IARC MONOGRAPHS

ON THE

EVALUATION OF THE CARCINOGENIC RISK

OF CHEMICALS TO MAN:

Some Carbamates, Thiocarbamates and Carbazides

Volume 12

This publication represents the views of an
IARC Working Group on the
Evaluation of the Carcinogenic Risk of Chemicals to Man
which met in Lyon,
9-15 June 1976

IARC WORKING GROUP ON THE EVALUATION OF THE CARCINOGENIC RISK OF CHEMICALS
TO MAN: SOME CARBAMATES, THIOCARBAMATES AND CARBAZIDES

Lyon, 9–15 June 1976

Members[1]

Dr R.R. Bates, Associate Commissioner for Science, US Food and Drug
Administration, 200 C Street SW, Washington DC 20204, USA (*Chairman*)

Professor E. Boyland, TUC Institute of Occupational Health, London School
of Hygiene and Tropical Medicine, Keppel Street, London WC1E 7HT, UK

Dr G.J. van Esch, Head, Laboratory for Toxicology, Rijks Instituut voor de
Volksgezondheid, Antonie van Leeuwenhoeklaan 9, Bilthoven, The Netherlands
(*Vice-Chairman*)

Dr D.E. Hathway, Senior Research Scientist, Central Toxicology Laboratory,
Imperial Chemical Industries Limited, Alderley Park, Cheshire SK10 4TJ,
UK

Dr W. Lijinsky, Frederick Cancer Research Centre, PO Box B, Frederick,
Maryland 21701, USA

Professor U. Mohr, Director, Abteilung für Experimentelle Pathologie,
Medizinische Hochschule Hannover, Karl Wiechert Allee 9, 3 Hannover 61,
FRG

Dr S.D. Murphy, Associate Professor of Toxicology, School of Public Health,
Department of Physiology, Harvard University, 665 Huntington Avenue,
Boston, Massachusetts 02115, USA

Dr V.B. Okulov, N. Petrov Research Institute of Oncology, 68 Leningradskaya
Street, Pesochny-2, Leningrad 188646, USSR

Dr C. Ramel, Stockholms Universitet, Wallenberglaboratoriet, Lilla Frescati,
S-104 05 Stockholm 50, Sweden

Dr B. Teichmann, Akademie der Wissenschaften der DDR, Zentralinstitut für
Krebsforschung, Lindenberger Weg 80, 1115 Berlin-Buch, GDR

Dr B. Terracini, Istituto di Anatomia e Istologia Patologica dell'Università
di Torino, Via Santena 7, 10126 Turin, Italy

---

[1]Unable to attend: Professor F.H. Sobels, Department of Radiation
Genetics and Chemical Mutagenesis, State University of Leiden,
Wassenaarseweg 72, Leiden 2405, The Netherlands

Invited Guests

Dr B. Hildebrand, Toxicology Department, BASF Aktiengesellschaft,
Brunckstrasse 60, D-6700 Ludwigshafen, FRG

Dr O.H. Johnson, Senior Industrial Economist, Chemical-Environmental
Program, Chemical Industries Center, Stanford Research Institute,
Menlo Park, California 94025, USA (*Rapporteur sections 2.1 and 2.2*)

Dr V. von Schuller-Götzburg, Manager, Chemical Information Services - Europe,
Stanford Research Institute, Pelikanstrasse 37, 8001 Zürich, Switzerland

Mrs M.-T. van der Venne, Commission of the European Communities, Health and
Safety Directorate, Building Jean Monnet A2/115, Avenue Alcide-de-Gasperi,
Kirchberg, Luxembourg, Great Duchy of Luxembourg

Representative from the National Cancer Institute

Dr J.A. Cooper, Deputy Associate Director, Carcinogenesis Program, Division
of Cancer Cause and Treatment, National Cancer Institute, Bethesda,
Maryland 20014, USA

Secretariat

Dr C. Agthe, Unit of Chemical Carcinogenesis (*Secretary*)

Dr H. Bartsch, Unit of Chemical Carcinogenesis (*Rapporteur section 3.2*)

Dr L. Griciute, Chief, Unit of Environmental Carcinogens

Dr R. Montesano, Unit of Chemical Carcinogenesis (*Rapporteur section 3.1*)

Mrs C. Partensky, Unit of Chemical Carcinogenesis (*Technical editor*)

Mrs I. Peterschmitt, Unit of Chemical Carcinogenesis, WHO, Geneva
(*Bibliographic researcher*)

Dr V. Ponomarkov, Unit of Chemical Carcinogenesis

Dr R. Saracci, Unit of Epidemiology and Biostatistics (*Rapporteur
section 3.3*)

Dr L. Tomatis, Chief, Unit of Chemical Carcinogenesis (*Head of the
Programme*)

Dr G. Vettorazzi, Food Additives Unit, WHO, Geneva

Mr E.A. Walker, Unit of Environmental Carcinogens (*Rapporteur sections
1 and 2.3*)

Mrs E. Ward, Montignac, France (*Editor*)

Mr J.D. Wilbourn, Unit of Chemical Carcinogenesis (*Co-secretary*)

Note to the reader

Every effort is made to present the monographs as accurately as possible without unduly delaying their publication. Nevertheless, mistakes have occurred and are still likely to occur. In the interest of all users of these monographs, readers are requested to communicate any errors observed to the Unit of Chemical Carcinogenesis of the International Agency for Research on Cancer, Lyon, France, in order that these can be included in corrigenda which will appear in subsequent volumes.

Since the monographs are not intended to be a review of the literature and contain only data considered relevant by the Working Group, it is not possible for the reader to determine whether a certain study was considered or not. However, research workers who are aware of important published data that may change the evaluation are requested to make them available to the above-mentioned address, in order that they can be considered for a possible re-evaluation by a future Working Group.

CONTENTS

BACKGROUND AND PURPOSE OF THE IARC PROGRAMME ON THE EVALUATION OF THE CARCINOGENIC RISK OF CHEMICALS TO MAN

The International Agency for Research on Cancer (IARC) initiated in 1971 a programme to evaluate the carcinogenic risk of chemicals to man. This programme was supported by a Resolution of the Governing Council at its Ninth Session concerning the role of IARC in providing government authorities with expert, independent scientific opinion on environmental carcinogenesis.

In view of the importance of the project and in order to expedite production of monographs, the National Cancer Institute of the United States has provided IARC with additional funds for this purpose.

The objective of the programme is to elaborate and publish in the form of monographs critical reviews of carcinogenicity and related data in the light of the present state of knowledge, with the final aim of evaluating the data in terms of possible human risk, and at the same time to indicate where additional research efforts are needed.

SCOPE OF THE MONOGRAPHS

The monographs summarize the evidence for the carcinogenicity of individual chemicals and other relevant information on the basis of data compiled, reviewed and evaluated by a Working Group of experts. No recommendations are given concerning preventive measures or legislation, since these matters depend on risk-benefit evaluations, which seem best made by individual governments and/or international agencies such as WHO and ILO.

Since 1971, when the programme was started, eleven volumes have been published[1-11]. As new data on chemicals for which monographs have already been prepared and new principles for evaluation become available, re-evaluations will be made at future meetings, and revised monographs will be published as necessary.

The monographs are distributed to international and governmental agencies, are available to industries and scientists dealing with these chemicals and are offered to any interested reader through their world-wide distribution as WHO publications. They also form the basis of advice from IARC on carcinogenesis from these substances.

MECHANISM FOR PRODUCING THE MONOGRAPHS

As a first step, a list of chemicals for possible consideration by the Working Group is established. IARC then collects pertinent references regarding physico-chemical characteristics, production and use*, occurrence and analysis and biological data** on these compounds. The material is summarized by an expert consultant or an IARC staff member, who prepares the first draft, which in some cases is sent to another expert for comments. The drafts are circulated to all members of the Working Group about one month before the meeting. During the meeting, further additions to and deletions from the data are agreed upon, and a final version of comments and evaluation on each compound is adopted.

Priority for the preparation of monographs

Priority is given mainly to chemicals belonging to particular chemical groups and for which there is at least some suggestion of carcinogenicity from observations in animals and/or man and evidence of human exposure. However, *the inclusion of a particular compound in a volume does not necessarily mean that it is considered to be carcinogenic. Equally, the fact that a substance has not yet been considered does not imply that it is without carcinogenic hazard.*

Data on which the evaluation is based

With regard to the biological data, only published articles and papers already accepted for publication are reviewed. The monographs are not intended to be a full review of the literature, and they contain only data considered relevant by the Working Group. Research workers who are aware

---

*Data provided by Chemical Information Services, Stanford Research Institute, Menlo Park, California, USA

**In the collection of original data reference was made to the series of publications 'Survey of Compounds which have been Tested for Carcinogenic Activity'[12-17].

of important data (published or accepted for publication) that may influence the evaluation are invited to make them available to the Unit of Chemical Carcinogenesis of the International Agency for Research on Cancer, Lyon, France.

The Working Group

The tasks of the Working Group are five-fold: (1) to ascertain that all data have been collected; (2) to select the data relevant for the evaluation; (3) to determine whether the data, as summarized, will enable the reader to follow the reasoning of the committee; (4) to judge the significance of results of experimental and epidemiological studies; and (5) to make an evaluation.

The members of the Working Group who participated in the consideration of particular substances are listed at the beginning of each publication. The members serve in their individual capacities as scientists and not as representatives of their governments or of any organization with which they are affiliated.

GENERAL PRINCIPLES FOR THE EVALUATION

These general principles for evaluation of carcinogenicity were elaborated by previous Working Groups and also applied to the substances covered in this volume.

Terminology

The term 'chemical carcinogenesis' in its widely accepted sense is used to indicate the induction or enhancement of neoplasia by chemicals. It is recognized that, in the strict etymological sense, this term means the induction of cancer; however, common usage has led to its employment to denote the induction of various types of neoplasms. The terms tumourigen 'oncogen' and 'blastomogen' have all been used synonymously with carcinogen although occasionally 'tumourigen' has been used specifically to denote the induction of benign tumours.

Response to carcinogens

In general, no distinction is made between the induction of tumours and the enhancement of tumour incidence, although it is noted that there may be fundamental differences in mechanisms that will eventually be elucidated. The response of experimental animals to a carcinogen may take several forms: a significant increase in the incidence of one or more of the same types of neoplasms as found in control animals; the occurrence of types of neoplasms not observed in control animals; and/or a decreased latent period for the production of neoplasms as compared with that in control animals.

Purity of the compounds tested

In any evaluation of biological data with respect to a possible carcinogenic risk, particular attention must be paid to the purity of the chemicals tested and to their stability under conditions of storage or administration. Information on purity and stability is given, when available, in the monographs.

Qualitative aspects

In many instances, both benign and malignant tumours are induced by chemical carcinogens. There are so far few recorded instances in which only benign tumours are induced by chemicals that have been studied extensively. Their occurrence in experimental systems has been taken to indicate the possibility of an increased risk of malignant tumours also.

In experimental carcinogenesis, the type of cancer seen may be the same as that recorded in human studies, e.g., bladder cancer in man, monkeys, dogs and hamsters after administration of 2-naphthylamine. In other instances, however, a chemical may induce other types of neoplasms at different sites in various species, e.g., benzidine induces hepatic carcinoma in rats but bladder carcinoma in man.

Quantitative aspects

Dose-response studies are important in the evaluation of human and animal carcinogenesis: the confidence with which a carcinogenic effect can be established is strengthened by the observation of an increasing

12

incidence of neoplasms with increasing exposure. In addition, such studies form the only basis on which a minimal effective dose can be established, allowing some comparison with data for human exposure.

Comparisons of compounds with regard to potency can only be made when the substances have been tested simultaneously.

Animal data in relation to the evaluation of risk to man

At the present time no attempt can be made to interpret the animal data directly in terms of human risk, since no objective criteria are available to do so. The critical assessments of the validity of the animal data given in these monographs are intended to assist national and/or international authorities in making decisions concerning preventive measures or legislation. In this connection attention is drawn to WHO recommendations in relation to food additives[18], drugs[19] and occupational carcinogens[20].

Evidence of human carcinogenicity

Evaluation of the carcinogenic risk to man of suspected environmental agents rests on purely observational studies. Such studies must cover a sufficient variation in levels of human exposure to allow a meaningful relationship between cancer incidence and exposure to a given chemical to be established. Difficulties arise in isolating the effects of individual agents, however, since people are usually exposed to multiple carcinogens.

The initial suggestion of a relationship between an agent and disease often comes from case reports of patients with similar exposures. Variations and time trends in regional or national cancer incidences, or their correlation with regional or national 'exposure' levels, may also provide valuable insights. Such observations by themselves, however, cannot in most circumstances be regarded as conclusive evidence of carcinogenicity.

The most satisfactory epidemiological method is to compare the cancer risk (adjusted for age, sex and other confounding variables) among groups or cohorts, or among individuals exposed to various levels of the agent in question, and among control groups not so exposed. Ideally, this is accomplished directly, by following such groups forward in time (prospectively) to determine time relationships, dose-response relationships and other aspects of cancer induction. Large cohorts and long observation periods are required to provide sufficient cases for a statistically valid comparison.

An alternative to prospective investigation is to assemble cohorts from past records and to evaluate their subsequent morbidity or mortality by means of medical histories and death certificates. Such occupational carcinogens as nickel, β-naphthylamine, asbestos and benzidine have been confirmed by this method.

Another method is to compare the past exposures of a defined group of cancer cases with those of control samples from the hospital or general population. This does not provide an absolute measure of carcinogenic risk but can indicate the relative risks associated with different levels of exposure.

Indirect means (e.g., interviews or tissue residues) of measuring exposures which may have commenced many years before can constitute a major source of error. Nevertheless, such 'case-control' studies can often isolate one factor from several suspected agents and can thus indicate which substance should be followed up by cohort studies.

EXPLANATORY NOTES ON THE MONOGRAPHS

In sections 1, 2 and 3 of each monograph, except for minor remarks, the data are recorded as given by the author, whereas the comments by the Working Group are given in section 4, headed 'Comments on Data Reported and Evaluation'.

Chemical and Physical Data (section 1)

The Chemical Abstracts Registry Serial Number and the latest Chemical Abstracts Name are recorded in this section, together with other synonyms and trade names.

Chemical and physical properties include, in particular, data that might be relevant to carcinogenicity (for example, lipid solubility) and those that concern identification. Data for which no reference is given are usually taken from standard reference books such as the *Merck Index*[21] or the *Handbook of Chemistry and Physics*[22]. All chemical data in this section refer to the pure substance, unless otherwise specified.

14

Production, Use, Occurrence and Analysis (section 2)

The purpose of this section is to indicate the extent of possible human exposure. With regard to data on production, use and occurrence, IARC has collaborated with the Stanford Research Institute, USA, with the support of the National Cancer Institute of the USA. Since cancer is a delayed toxic effect, past use and production data are also provided.

The United States, Europe and Japan are reasonably representative industrialized areas of the world, and if data on production or use are available from these countries they are reported. It should *not*, however, be inferred that these nations are the sole or even the major sources of any individual chemical.

Production data are obtained from both governmental and trade publications in the three geographic areas. Information on use and occurrence is obtained by a comprehensive review of published data, complemented by direct contact with manufacturers of the chemical in questions. In an effort to provide estimates of production in some European countries, the Stanford Research Institute in Zurich sent questionnaires to certain European companies thought to produce carbamates, thiocarbamates and carbazides. The replies have been included in the individual monographs.

Statements concerning regulations in some countries are mentioned as examples only. They may not reflect the most recent situation, since such legislation is in a constant state of change; nor should it be taken to imply that other countries do not have similar regulations. In the case of drugs, mention of the therapeutic uses of such chemicals does not necessarily represent presently accepted therapeutic indications, nor does it imply judgement as to their clinical efficacy.

The purpose of the section on analysis is to give the reader an indication of methods available in the literature. No attempt is made to evaluate the methods quoted.

Biological Data Relevant to the Evaluation of Carcinogenic Risk to Man (section 3)

The monographs are not intended to consider all reported studies. Some studies were purposely omitted (a) because they were inadequate, as judged from previously described criteria[23-26] (e.g., too short a duration, too few animals, poor survival or too small a dose); (b) because they only confirmed findings which have already been fully described; or (c) because they were judged irrelevant for the purpose of the evaluation. However, in certain cases, reference is made to studies which did not meet established criteria of adequacy, particularly when this information was considered a useful supplement to other reports or when it was the only data available. Their inclusion does not, however, imply acceptance of the adequacy of their experimental design.

In general, the data recorded in this section are summarized as given by the author; however, certain shortcomings of reporting or of experimental design that were commented upon by the Working Group are given in square brackets.

Carcinogenicity and related studies in animals: Mention is made of all routes of administration by which the compound has been adequately tested and of all species in which relevant tests have been carried out. In most cases, animal strains are given; general characteristics of mouse strains have been reported in a recent review[27]. Quantitative data are given to indicate the order of magnitude of the effective doses. In general, the doses are reported as they appear in the original paper; sometimes conversions have been made for better comparison.

Other relevant biological data: Some LD_{50}'s are given, and other data on toxicity are included, when considered relevant. The metabolic data included is restricted to studies showing the metabolic fate of the chemical in animals and man, and comparisons of animal and human data are made when possible. Other metabolic information (e.g., absorption, storage and excretion) is given when the Working Group considered that it would be useful for the reader to have a better understanding of the fate of the compound in the body. When the carcinogenicity of known metabolites has been tested, this also is reported.

Mutagenicity data are also included; the reasons for including them and the principles adopted by the Working Group for their selection are outlined below.

Many, but not all, mutagens are carcinogens and *vice versa*; the exact level of correlation is still under investigation. Nevertheless, practical use may be made of the available mutagenicity test procedures that combine microbial, mammalian or other animal cell systems as genetic targets with an *in vitro* or *in vivo* metabolic activation system. The results of relatively rapid and inexpensive mutagenicity tests on non-human organisms may help to pre-screen chemicals and may also aid in the selection of the most relevant animal species in which to carry out long-term carcinogenicity tests on these chemicals.

The role of genetic alterations in chemical carcinogenesis is not yet fully understood, and therefore consideration must be given to a variety of changes. Although nuclear DNA has been defined as the main cellular target for the induction of genetic changes, other relevant targets have been recognized, e.g., mitochondrial DNA, enzymes involved in DNA synthesis, repair and recombination, and the spindle apparatus. Tests to detect the genetic activity of chemicals, including gene mutation, structural and numerical chromosomal changes and mitotic recombination, are available for non-human models; but not all such tests can be applied at present to human cells.

Ideally, an appropriate mutagenicity test system would include the full metabolic competency of the intact human. Since the development or application of such a system appears to be impossible, a battery of test systems is necessary in order to establish the mutagenic potential of chemicals. There are many genetic indicators and metabolic activation systems available for detecting mutagenic activity; they all, however, have individual advantages and limitations.

Since many chemicals require metabolism to an active form, test systems which do not take this into account may fail to reveal the full range of genetic damage. Furthermore, since some reactive metabolites with a limited lifespan may fail to reach or to react with the genetic indicator, either because they are further metabolized to inactive compounds or because they react with other cellular constituents, mutagenicity tests in intact animals may give false negative results.

It is difficult in the present state of knowledge to select specific mutagenicity tests as being the most appropriate for the pre-screening of substances for possible carcinogenic activity. However, greater reliance may be placed on data obtained from those test systems which (a) permit identification of the nature of induced genetic changes, and (b) demonstrate that the changes are transmitted to subsequent generations. Mutagenicity tests using organisms that are well-understood genetically, e.g., *Escherichia coli*, *Salmonella typhimurium*, *Saccharomyces* and *Drosophila*, meet these requirements.

Although a correlation has often been observed between the ability of a chemical to cause chromosome breakage and its ability to induce gene mutation, data on chromosomal breakage alone do not provide adequate evidence for mutagenicity, and therefore less weight should be given to pre-screening that is based on the use of peripheral leucocyte cultures.

Because of the complexity of factors that can contribute to reproductive failure, as well as the insensitivity of the method, the dominant lethal test in the mammal does not provide reliable data on mutagenicity.

A large-scale systematic screening of compounds to assess a correlation between mutagenicity and carcinogenicity has so far been carried out only with the bacterial/mammalian liver microsome system. Notwithstanding the demonstration of the mutagenicity of many known carcinogens to *Salmonella typhimurium* in the presence of liver microsomal systems, the possibility of false-negative and false-positive results must not be overlooked. False-negatives might arise as a consequence of mutagen specificity or from failure to achieve optimal conditions for activation *in vitro*. Alternative test systems must be used if there appear to be substantial reasons for suspecting that a chemical which is apparently non-mutagenic in a bacterial test system may nevertheless be potentially carcinogenic. Conversely, some chemicals found to be mutagenic in this test may not in fact have mutagenic activity in other systems.

18

For more detailed information, see references 28-35.

Observations in man: Case reports of cancer and epidemiological studies are summarized in this section.

Comments on Data Reported and Evaluation (section 4)

This section gives the critical view of the Working Group on the data reported. It should be read in conjunction with the 'General Remarks on Carbamates, Thiocarbamates and Carbazides', p. 23.

Animal data: The animal species mentioned are those in which the carcinogenicity of the substances was clearly demonstrated, irrespective of the route of administration. The route of administration used in experimental animals that is similar to the possible human exposure (ingestion, inhalation and skin exposure) is given particular mention. In most cases, tumour sites are also indicated.

Experiments involving a possible action of the vehicle or a physical effect of the agent, such as in studies by subcutaneous injection or bladder implanation, are included; however, the results of such tests require careful consideration, particularly if they are the only ones raising a suspicion of carcinogenicity. If the substance has produced tumours after pre-natal exposure or in single-dose experiments, this also is indicated. This sub-section should be read in the light of comments made in the section, 'Animal Data in Relation to the Evaluation of Risk to Man' of this introduction.

Human data: In some cases, a brief statement is made on possible human exposure. The significance of epidemiological studies and case reports is discussed, and the data are interpreted in terms of possible human risk.

References

1. IARC (1972) *IARC Monographs on the Evaluation of Carcinogenic Risk of Chemicals to Man*, 1, Lyon

2. IARC (1973) *IARC Monographs on the Evaluation of Carcinogenic Risk of Chemicals to Man*, 2, *Some Inorganic and Organometallic Compounds*, Lyon

3. IARC (1973) *IARC Monographs on the Evaluation of Carcinogenic Risk of Chemicals to Man*, 3, *Certain Polycyclic Aromatic Hydrocarbons and Heterocyclic Compounds*, Lyon

4. IARC (1974) *IARC Monographs on the Evaluation of Carcinogenic Risk of Chemicals to Man*, 4, *Some Aromatic Amines, Hydrazine and Related Substances, N-Nitroso Compounds and Miscellaneous Alkylating Agents*, Lyon

5. IARC (1974) *IARC Monographs on the Evaluation of Carcinogenic Risk of Chemicals to Man*, 5, *Some Organochlorine Pesticides*, Lyon

6. IARC (1974) *IARC Monographs on the Evaluation of Carcinogenic Risk of Chemicals to Man*, 6, *Sex Hormones*, Lyon

7. IARC (1974) *IARC Monographs on the Evaluation of Carcinogenic Risk of Chemicals to Man*, 7, *Some Anti-thyroid and Related Substances, Nitrofurans and Industrial Chemicals*, Lyon

8. IARC (1975) *IARC Monographs on the Evaluation of Carcinogenic Risk of Chemicals to Man*, 8, *Some Aromatic Azo Compounds*, Lyon

9. IARC (1975) *IARC Monographs on the Evaluation of Carcinogenic Risk of Chemicals to Man*, 9, *Some Aziridines, N-, S- and O-Mustards and Selenium*, Lyon

10. IARC (1976) *IARC Monographs on the Evaluation of Carcinogenic Risk of Chemicals to Man*, 10, *Some Naturally Occurring Substances*, Lyon

11. IARC (1976) *IARC Monographs on the Evaluation of Carcinogenic Risk of Chemicals to Man*, 11, *Cadmium, Nickel, Some Epoxides, Miscellaneous Industrial Chemicals and General Considerations on Volatile Anaesthetics*, Lyon

12. Hartwell, J.L. (1951) *Survey of Compounds which have been Tested for Carcinogenic Activity*, Washington DC, US Government Printing Office (Public Health Service Publication No. 149)

13. Shubik, P. & Hartwell, J.L. (1957) *Survey of Compounds which have been Tested for Carcinogenic Activity*, Washington DC, US Government Printing Office (Public Health Service Publication No. 149: Supplement 1)

14.   Shubik, P. & Hartwell, J.L. (1969) Survey of Compounds which have
       been Tested for Carcinogenic Activity, Washington DC, US
       Government Printing Office (Public Health Service Publication
       No. 149: Supplement 2)

15.   Carcinogenesis Program National Cancer Institute (1971) Survey of
       Compounds which have been Tested for Carcinogenic Activity,
       Washington DC, US Government Printing Office (Public Health
       Service Publication No. 149: 1968-1969)

16.   Carcinogenesis Program National Cancer Institute (1973) Survey of
       Compounds which have been Tested for Carcinogenic Activity,
       Washington DC, US Government Printing Office (Public Health
       Service Publication No. 149: 1961-1967)

17.   Carcinogenesis Program National Cancer Institute (1974) Survey of
       Compounds which have been Tested for Carcinogenic Activity,
       Washington DC, US Government Printing Office (Public Health
       Service Publication No. 149: 1970-1971)

18.   WHO (1961) Fifth Report of the Joint FAO/WHO Expert Committee on
       Food Additives. Evaluation of carcinogenic hazard of food
       additives. Wld Hlth Org. techn. Rep. Ser., No. 220, pp. 5, 18, 19

19.   WHO (1969) Report of a WHO Scientific Group. Principles for the
       testing and evaluation of drugs for carcinogenicity. Wld Hlth
       Org. techn. Rep. Ser., No. 426, pp. 19, 21, 22

20.   WHO (1964) Report of a WHO Expert Committee. Prevention of cancer.
       Wld Hlth Org. techn. Rep. Ser., No. 276, pp. 29, 30

21.   Stecher, P.G., ed. (1968) The Merck Index, 8th ed., Rahway, NJ,
       Merck & Co.

22.   Weast, R.C., ed. (1975) CRC Handbook of Chemistry and Physics,
       56th ed., Cleveland, Ohio, Chemical Rubber Co.

23.   WHO (1958) Second Report of the Joint FAO/WHO Expert Committee on
       Food Additives. Procedures for the testing of intentional
       food additives to establish their safety for use. Wld Hlth Org.
       techn. Rep. Ser., No. 144

24.   WHO (1961) Fifth Report of the Joint FAO/WHO Expert Committee on
       Food Additives. Evaluation of carcinogenic hazard of food
       additives. Wld Hlth Org. techn. Rep. Ser., No. 220

25.   WHO (1967) Scientific Group. Procedures for investigating intentional
       and unintentional food additives. Wld Hlth Org. techn. Rep. Ser.,
       No. 348

26.   Berenblum, I., ed. (1969) Carcinogenicity testing. UICC techn. Rep.
       Ser., 2

27. Committee on Standardized Genetic Nomenclature for Mice (1972)
     Standardized nomenclature for inbred strains of mice. Fifth
     listing. Cancer Res., 32, 1609-1646

28. Bartsch, H. & Grover, P.L. (1976) Chemical carcinogenesis and muta-
     genesis. In: Symington, T. & Carter, R.L., eds, Scientific
     Foundations of Oncology, Vol. IX, Chemical Carcinogenesis,
     London, Heinemann Medical Books Ltd, pp. 334-342

29. Holländer, A., ed. (1971) Chemical Mutagens: Principles and Methods
     for Their Detection, Vols 1-3, New York, Plenum Press

30. Montesano, R. & Tomatis, L., eds (1974) Chemical Carcinogenesis
     Essays, Lyon, IARC (IARC Scientific Publications No. 10)

31. Ramel, C., ed. (1973) Evaluation of genetic risks of environmental
     chemicals: report of a symposium held at Skokloster, Sweden,
     1972. Ambio Special Report, No. 3

32. Stoltz, D.R., Poirier, L.A., Irving, C.C., Stich, H.F., Weisburger,
     J.H. & Grice, H.C. (1974) Evaluation of short-term tests for
     carcinogenicity. Toxicol. appl. Pharmacol., 29, 157-180

33. WHO (1974) Report of WHO Scientific Group. Assessment of the
     carcinogenicity and mutagenicity of chemicals. Wld Hlth Org.
     techn. Rep. Ser., No. 546

34. Montesano, R., Bartsch, H. & Tomatis, L., eds (1975) Screening Tests
     in Chemical Carcinogenesis, Lyon, IARC (IARC Scientific Publi-
     cations No. 12)

35. Committee 17 (1975) Environmental mutagenic hazards. Science, 187,
     503-514

GENERAL REMARKS ON CARBAMATES, THIOCARBAMATES AND CARBAZIDES

In this volume of monographs, a number of carbamate esters, dialkyl-dithiocarbamates, ethylene bisdithiocarbamates and carbazides are considered, which are or have been produced and for which a carcinogenic effect or a suspicion of carcinogenicity has been reported.

The Working Group was aware of unpublished data concerning some of these compounds. However, in view of the principle followed in these monographs not to use data which are unavailable to the reader, such information was not considered by the Working Group. The members expressed concern over the long delay which sometimes occurs in the publication of experimental data.

For many of the chemicals considered in this volume (probably for more than in any other volume of this series), the Working Group was unable to make an evaluation of carcinogenicity: the data were either quantitatively or qualitatively inadequate. In addition, there was a consistent lack of epidemiological studies. In this context, it should be pointed out that the report which gave the results of the long-term testing of about 130 environmental chemicals (Innes *et al.*, 1969), upon which most of the evaluations of carcinogenicity of the compounds considered in this volume were based, was published in 1969. It is widely accepted that experimental data on the carcinogenicity of a chemical to which humans are exposed provide a good indication of the necessity for epidemiological studies; however, in spite of the fact that there is human exposure to most of the chemicals for which evidence of carcinogenicity or a suspicion of carcinogenicity was provided by this large study, discouragingly little epidemiological work has resulted in the seven years which have followed.

In so far as the experimental evidence is concerned, there are two main points which the Working Group would like to point out: (1) the chemicals considered in the monographs are selected among those for which not only some suspicion of carcinogenicity exists but for which, with a few exceptions, there is evidence of their use and production and social importance. Therefore, if the available data were insufficient for the Working Group to make an evaluation of a chemical considered in this series, further testing

of that chemical should be considered of high priority;   (2) it is
imperative that carcinogenicity testing be carried out following certain
basic requirements in order that the results can be properly evaluated.
The Agency is planning a discussion of protocols for testing which can be
agreed upon internationally, but there are already several publications
which give satisfactory information on the proper running of carcinogenicity
tests (Berenblum, 1969;   Golberg, 1974;   NCI, 1975).

The compounds considered in this volume are used as insecticides,
fungicides or herbicides, as accelerators in the vulcanization of rubber,
as drugs or as chemical intermediates in the manufacture of drugs,
pesticides or resins.

Surveys in the US, Europe and Japan have shown that a number of the
compounds are produced in quantities of up to several thousand kg per
annum;   production of some of the compounds may have been as high as
5 million kg in recent years, and for one (carbaryl) 24 million kg were
produced in the US in 1971. Although their occurrence in the environment
is thus to be expected, there is little data on their persistence and
breakdown.

As mentioned above, a substantial proportion of the biological information related to carcinogenicity in experimental animals included in the
present series of monographs derives from a large-scale study of about
130 chemicals. In this study, each chemical was tested both by long-term
feeding and by single subcutaneous injection in two hybrid strains of mice.
A partial summary of the results was published in 1969 (Innes *et al.*, 1969),
and the details of each experiment are available in a separate publication
(NTIS, 1968). In both reports, results for each strain, sex and route of
administration are given as numbers of animals developing tumours and not
as numbers of tumours found at each site;   nor is the age at death of
tumour-bearing mice given. Therefore, precise analytical methods, such as
the construction of lifetime tables, could not be used, and the statistical
significance of the results has been established using the χ^2 method,
systematically introducing Yates' continuity correction (even when the
authors may have used a different procedure). Results obtained from
animals receiving the same compound by different routes or belonging to

24

different strains were evaluated separately by the Working Group; however, in some cases, the statistical significance was established by combining results obtained in the two sexes of the same strain receiving the same treatment.

There have been reports that many N-alkylureas or N-alkylcarbamates (and thiocarbamates) react with nitrite under mildly acidic conditions to form N-nitroso compounds (Mirvish, 1975; Sen *et al.*, 1974). Nitrite is formed by bacterial reduction of nitrate, which is accumulated to significantly high concentrations in some vegetables (e.g., spinach and beets) on standing in air, especially after cooking (Ashton, 1970; Phillips, 1968). The 6-10 ppm nitrite found in human saliva result from reduction of nitrate by bacteria in the mouth (Tannenbaum *et al.*, 1974). A major source of nitrite is cured meats, in which concentrations of up to 100 ppm are common (Ashton, 1970). Table I lists several alkylureas, alkylcarbamates and thiocarbamates that have been shown to react with nitrite in chemical systems. The formation of N-nitrosodimethylamine by the action of microorganisms in sewage and soil containing 0.1% thiram has been reported to occur under experimental conditions (Ayanaba *et al.*, 1973). N-Nitroso compounds derived similarly from other carbamate pesticides could also occur in the environment.

It is not known to what extent the formation of N-nitroso derivatives by reaction of carbamate pesticides with nitrite, as shown in chemical systems, could take place in man *in vivo*. Extrapolation of chemical findings to the significance of such reactions in man is complicated by several factors, including drastic differences in the concentrations of the reactants, differences in pH and the possible presence of accelerators and inhibitors of the reaction.

The N-nitrosodialkylamines (N-nitrosodiethyl- and N-nitrosodimethylamines), formed from dialkylthiocarbamate pesticides and nitrite, are potent carcinogens and mutagens. The N-nitroso derivatives of several N-alkylcarbamates and N-alkylureas have given rise to malignant tumours in experimental animals at small doses; these include N-nitrosobenzthiazuron (Ungerer *et al.*, 1974) and N-nitrosocarbaryl which induce tumours in rats (Eisenbrand *et al.*, 1975, 1976; Lijinsky & Taylor, 1976). N-Nitrosocarbaryl has also

Table I

Reactions of alkylureas, alkylcarbamates and thiocarbamates with nitrite

Compound	*N*-Nitroso derivative formed
Benzthiazuron (*N*-(2-benzothiazolyl)-*N'*- methylurea)	*N*-Nitrosobenzthiazuron (Eisenbrand *et al.*, 1974b; Ungerer *et al.*, 1974)
Carbaryl	*N*-Nitrosocarbaryl (Eisenbrand *et al.*, 1974b; Elespuru & Lijinsky, 1973)
Disulfiram	*N*-Nitrosodiethylamine (Lijinsky *et al.*, 1972)
Dulcin	*N*-Nitrosodulcin (Mirvish, 1975)
Fenuron (1,1-dimethyl-3-phenylurea)	*N*-Nitrosodimethylamine (Mirvish, 1975)
Ferbam	*N*-Nitrosodimethylamine (Sen *et al.*, 1974)
Propoxur (2-isopropoxyphenyl-*N*- methylcarbamate)	*N*-Nitrosopropoxur (Eisenbrand *et al.*, 1974b)
Thiram	*N*-Nitrosodimethylamine (Egert & Greim, 1976; Sen *et al.*, 1974)
Ziram	*N*-Nitrosodimethylamine (Eisenbrand *et al.*, 1974a,b; Sen *et al.*, 1974)

induced malignant transformation in Balb/3T3 mouse cells in culture (Quarles & Tennant, 1975).

Many of the compounds considered in the present volume, e.g., the *N*-methylcarbamates, carbaryl and zectran, the *N,N*-diisopropylthiocarbamate, diallate, and the dithiocarbamates, zineb and ziram, cause central nervous system malfunction under conditions of severe poisoning (Best & Murray, 1962; Hodge *et al.*, 1956; Komarova & Zotkina, 1971; Pestova, 1966; Richardson & Batteese, 1973; Ryazanova *et al.*, 1972). The *N*-methylcarbamates, carbaryl and zectran, have been shown to inhibit acetylcholinesterase activity (for references, see individual monographs).

Hydrolytic fission is the principal primary metabolic pathway for the simple ester carbamates and dimethylcarbamoyl chloride (von Hey *et al.*, 1974; Queen, 1967), and this biotransformation applies to a lesser extent to the aromatic *N*-methylcarbamates, carbaryl and zectran, the *N*-phenylcarbamates, chloropropham and propham, and the *N*-phenyldialkylurea, monuron. In addition, while ring hydroxylation is a feature of the metabolism of the aromatic *N*-methylcarbamates and of the *N*-phenylcarbamates, oxidative N-dealkylation takes place with the *N*-phenyldialkylurea; but *N*-phenylcarbamates undergo oxidation of the isopropyl group (without dealkylation) (for references, see individual monographs). Epoxidation and subsequent ring fission by hydrolysis (Sullivan *et al.*, 1972) and by reaction with glutathione (Bend *et al.*, 1971) are important biotransformations of carbaryl. In the N-dealkylation pathway, carbaryl (Dorough & Casida, 1964; Dorough *et al.*, 1963; Leeling & Casida, 1966) and zectran (Oonnithan & Casida, 1966) afford reactive methylolamides, and carbaryl, like the simple ester carbamates, also undergoes N-hydroxylation (Locke, 1972).

Reductive fission of the disulphide bond of the tetraalkylthiuram disulphides, disulfiram (Domar *et al.*, 1949) and thiram, occurs *in vivo*, and the resulting dialkyldithiocarbamates have a metabolic pathway in common with those belonging to the sodium (Strömme, 1965), iron (ferbam) and zinc (ziram) salts (Hodgson *et al.*, 1975), e.g., fission of dialkyldithiocarbamate into carbon disulphide and dialkylamine and N-glucuronidation of the dialkyl-dithiocarbamate itself. The ethylene bisdithiocarbamates, maneb and zineb, undergo other metabolic changes, including hydrolytic reactions, rearrangements, ring fission with extrusion of carbon disulphide and ring closure (Seidler *et al.*, 1970; Truhaut *et al.*, 1973).

The fact that dimethylcarbamoyl chloride behaves as a direct-acting carcinogen (Van Duuren *et al.*, 1972) is consistent with the production *in vivo* of the corresponding carbonium ion, which reacts with nucleophiles (Hall & Lueck, 1963). Ethylenethiourea, which produces thyroid carcinomas in rats and liver-cell tumours in mice after its oral administration (IARC, 1974), is formed from ethylenebisdithiocarbamates, such as maneb and zineb, both by metabolic processes and by cooking (Watts *et al.*, 1974).

Carbaryl, semicarbazide hydrochloride and *n*-propyl carbamate, the ethylenebisdithiocarbamates, maneb and zineb, the dialkyldithiocarbamate, ferbam, and the tetraalkylthiuram disulphide, thiram, are teratogenic in experimental animals (for references, see individual monographs).

Mutagenicity data on the carbamate compounds are limited and largely restricted to bacteria and plant material. It is possible that in higher plants some chemicals can undergo metabolic conversion into potent mutagens, as illustrated by the metabolism of atrazine (2-chloro-4-ethylamino-6-isopropylamine-*s*-triazine) in maize (Plewa & Gentile, 1975, 1976). Furthermore, the most pronounced genetic effect of some of the carbamates is inhibition of spindle-fibre formation, and this can most easily be studied in plants. Mutagenicity data in mammals or man were available for seven of the compounds considered.

Several bisdithiocarbamates are goitrogenic in laboratory animals, and there is some suggestion that this effect has occurred in men exposed to thiram. The relationship between goitrogenicity and carcinogenicity, and its practical consequences, have been dealt with elsewhere (IARC, 1974; WHO, 1974) but have not been fully elucidated.

From investigations in animals of the relationship between the structure of the dithiocarbamates and the occurrence of acetaldehyde in the blood after ingestion of ethanol, it appears that most of the alkyldithiocarbamates (e.g., ferbam and ziram) and thiuram sulphides (e.g., disulfiram and thiram) induce accumulation of acetaldehyde. The ethylenebisdithiocarbamates (e.g., zineb and maneb) had no effect on the acetaldehyde level in the blood.

On the whole, dithiocarbamates with a free H-atom on the N-atom did not show the dithiocarbamate-ethanol reaction in animals. There are indications that observations in studies of occupational health correspond with these results from animal studies (van Logten, 1972).

Of the compounds considered in this volume, disulfiram, dulcin, ethyl tellurac, ledate, monuron, semicarbazide hydrochloride and zectran are currently being tested for carcinogenicity in experimental animals, and an epidemiological survey is being carried out on dimethylcarbamoyl chloride (IARC Information Bulletin on the Survey of Chemicals Being Tested for Carcinogenicity, No. 6, 1976).

Several other carbamate compounds (listed below) inhibit tumour growth but are also carcinogenic in animals. Since there was no available evidence of past or current human exposure to these compounds, monographs on them were not prepared: 1,1-diphenyl-2-propynyl-N-cyclohexyl carbamate (Harris et al., 1969); 1,1-bis(4-fluorophenyl)-2-propynyl-N-cycloheptyl carbamate and 1,1-bis(4-fluorophenyl)-2-propynyl-N-cyclooctyl carbamate (Harris et al., 1970); 1-(4-chlorophenyl)-1-phenyl-2-propynyl carbamate (Harris et al., 1972); and 1,4-bis(4-fluorophenyl)-2-propynyl-N-cyclooctyl carbamate (Weisburger et al., 1975).

Many other ureas and carbamate compounds, used as agricultural chemicals (Epstein & Legator, 1971; Kuhr & Dorough, 1976) and/or drugs (Stecher, 1968), are produced commercially, but no data on their carcinogenicity were available to the Working Group.

References

Ashton, M.R. (1970) The Occurrence of Nitrates and Nitrites in Foods, Leatherhead, Surrey, The British Food Manufacturing Industries Research Association

Ayanaba, A., Verstraete, W. & Alexander, M. (1973) Possible microbial contribution to nitrosamine formation in sewage and soil. J. nat. Cancer Inst., 50, 811-813

Bend, J.R., Holder, G.M., Protos, E. & Ryan, A.J. (1971) Water-soluble metabolites of carbaryl (1-naphthyl-N-methylcarbamate) in mouse liver preparations and in the rat. Austr. J. biol. Sci., 24, 535-546

Berenblum, I., ed. (1969) Carcinogenicity testing. UICC techn. Rep. Ser., 2

Best, E.M., Jr & Murray, B.L. (1962) Observations on workers exposed to sevin insecticide: a preliminary report. J. occup. Med., 4, 507-517

Domar, G., Fredga, A. & Linderholm, H. (1949) A method for quantitative determination of tetraethylthiuram disulphide (Antabuse, Abstimyl) and its reduced form, diethyldithiocarbamic acid, as found in excreta. Acta chem. scand., 3, 1441-1442

Dorough, H.W. & Casida, J.E. (1964) Nature of certain carbamate metabolites of the insecticide sevin. J. agric. Fd Chem., 12, 294-304

Dorough, H.W., Leeling, N.C. & Casida, J.E. (1963) Non-hydrolytic pathway in metabolism of N-methylcarbamate insecticides. Science, 140, 170-171

Egert, G. & Greim, H. (1976) Formation of dimethylnitrosamine from chloroxuron, cycluron, dimefox and thiram in the presence of nitrite. Mutation Res., 38, 136-137

Eisenbrand, G., Ungerer, O. & Preussmann, R. (1974a) Rapid formation of carcinogenic N-nitrosamines by interaction of nitrite with fungicides derived from dithiocarbamic acid *in vitro* under simulated gastric conditions and *in vivo* in the rat stomach. Fd Cosmet. Toxicol., 12, 229-232

Eisenbrand, G., Ungerer, O. & Preussmann, R. (1974b) Formation of N-nitroso compounds from agricultural chemicals and nitrite. In: Bogovski, P. & Walker, E.A., eds, N-Nitroso Compounds in the Environment, Lyon, IARC (IARC Scientific Publications No. 9), pp. 71-74

Eisenbrand, G., Ungerer, O. & Preussmann, R. (1975) The reaction of nitrite with pesticides. II. Formation, chemical properties and carcinogenic activity of the N-nitroso derivative of N-methyl-1-naphthyl carbamate (carbaryl). Fd Cosmet. Toxicol., 13, 365-367

Eisenbrand, G., Schmähl, D. & Preussmann, R. (1976) Carcinogenicity in rats of high oral doses of *N*-nitrosocarbaryl, a nitrosated pesticide. Cancer Lett., 1, 281-284

Elespuru, R.K. & Lijinsky, W. (1973) The formation of carcinogenic nitroso compounds from nitrite and some types of agricultural chemicals. Fd Cosmet. Toxicol., 11, 807-817

Epstein, S.S. & Legator, M.S. (1971) The Mutagenicity of Pesticides - Concepts and Evaluation, Cambridge, Mass., MIT Press

Golberg, L., ed. (1974) Carcinogenicity Testing of Chemicals, Cleveland, Ohio, Chemical Rubber Co.

Hall, H.K., Jr & Lueck, C.H. (1963) The ionization mechanism for the hydrolysis of acyl chlorides. J. org. Chem., 28, 2818-2825

Harris, P.N., Gibson, W.R. & Dillard, R.D. (1969) Pluripotent oncogenicity of 1,1-diphenyl-2-propynyl *N*-cyclohexylcarbamate. I. Proc. Amer. Ass. Cancer Res., 10, 35

Harris, P.N., Gibson, W.R. & Dillard, R.D. (1970) The oncogenicity of two 1,1-diaryl-2-propynyl *N*-cycloalkylcarbamates. Cancer Res., 30, 2952-2954

Harris, P.N., Gibson, W.R. & Dillard, R.D. (1972) Oncogenicity of 1-(4-chlorophenyl)-1-phenyl-2-propynyl carbamate for rats. Toxicol. appl. Pharmacol., 21, 414-418

von Hey, W., Thiess, A.M. & Zeller, H. (1974) Zur Frage etwaiger Gesundheits-schädigungen bei der Herstellung und Verarbeitung von Dimethylcarbamin-säurechlorid. Zbl. Arbeitsmed., 24, 71-77

Hodge, H.C., Maynard, E.A., Downs, W.L., Coye, R.D., Jr & Steadman, L.T. (1956) Chronic oral toxicity of ferric dimethyldithiocarbamate (ferbam) and zinc dimethyldithiocarbamate (ziram). J. Pharmacol. exp. Ther., 118, 174-181

Hodgson, J.R., Hoch, J.C., Castles, T.R., Helton, D.O. & Lee, C.-C. (1975) Metabolism and disposition of ferbam in the rat. Toxicol. appl. Pharmacol., 33, 505-513

IARC (1974) IARC Monographs on the Evaluation of Carcinogenic Risk of Chemicals to Man, 7, Some Anti-thyroid and Related Substances, Nitro-furans and Industrial Chemicals, Lyon, pp. 23-26, 45-52

Innes, J.R.M., Ulland, B.M., Valerio, M.G., Petrucelli, L., Fishbein, L., Hart, E.R., Pallotta, A.J., Bates, R.R., Falk, H.L., Gart, J.J., Klein, M., Mitchell, I. & Peters, J. (1969) Bioassay of pesticides and industrial chemicals for tumorigenicity in mice: a preliminary note. J. nat. Cancer Inst., 42, 1101-1114

Komarova, A.A. & Zotkina, V.P. (1971) On the use of electromyography and certain indices of acetylcholine metabolism in evaluating the health status of workers engaged in the production of ziram. Gig. Tr. Prof. Zabol., 15, 17-20

Kuhr, R.J. & Dorough, H.W. (1976) Carbamate Insecticides: Chemistry, Biochemistry and Toxicology, Cleveland, Ohio, Chemical Rubber Co.

Leeling, N.C. & Casida, J.E. (1966) Metabolites of carbaryl (1-naphthyl-N-methylcarbamate) in mammals and enzymatic systems for their formation. J. agric. Fd Chem., 14, 281-290

Lijinsky, W. & Taylor, H.W. (1976) Carcinogenesis in Sprague-Dawley rats by N-nitroso-N-alkylcarbamate esters. Cancer Lett., 1, 275-279

Lijinsky, W., Conrad, E. & Van de Bogart, R. (1972) Carcinogenic nitrosamines formed by drug/nitrite interactions. Nature (Lond.), 239, 165-167

Locke, R.K. (1972) Thin-layer chromatography of 1-naphthyl-N-hydroxy-N-methyl carbamate and its application in two in vitro studies involving carbaryl. J. agric. Fd Chem., 20, 1078-1080

van Logten, M.J. (1972) De Dithiocarbamaat-Alcohol-Reactie bij de Rat, Terborg, The Netherlands, Bedrijf FA. Lammers

Mirvish, S.S. (1975) Formation of N-nitroso compounds: chemistry, kinetics and in vivo occurrence. Toxicol. appl. Pharmacol., 31, 325-351

NCI (National Cancer Institute) (1975) Guidelines for Carcinogen Bioassay in Small Rodents, Washington DC, US Department of Health, Education and Welfare

NTIS (National Technical Information Service) (1968) Evaluation of Carcinogenic, Teratogenic and Mutagenic Activities of Selected Pesticides and Industrial Chemicals, Vol. 1, Carcinogenic Study, Washington DC, US Department of Commerce

Oonnithan, E.S. & Casida, J.E. (1966) Metabolites of methyl- and dimethyl-carbamate insecticide chemicals as formed by rat liver microsomes. Bull. environm. Contam. Toxicol., 1, 59-69

Pestova, A.G. (1966) Toxicity of diptal and avadex. Gig. Toksikol. Pestits. Klin. Otravlenii, 4, 166-169

Phillips, W.E.J. (1968) Changes in the nitrate and nitrite contents of fresh and processed spinach during storage. J. agric. Fd Chem., 16, 88-91

Plewa, M.J. & Gentile, J.M. (1975) A maize-microbe bioassay for the detection of proximal mutagenicity of agricultural chemicals. Maize Genet. Coop. Newslett., 49, 40-43

Plewa, M.J. & Gentile, J.M. (1976) Mutagenicity of atrazine: a maize-microbe bioassay. Mutation Res., 38, 287-292

Quarles, J.M. & Tennant, R.W. (1975) Effects of nitrosocarbaryl on BALB/3T3 cells. Cancer Res., 35, 2637-2645

Queen, A. (1967) Kinetics of the hydrolysis of acyl chlorides in pure water. Canad. J. Chem., 45, 1619-1629

Richardson, E.M. & Batteese, R.I., Jr (1973) An incident of zectran poisoning. J. Maine med. Ass., 64, 158-159

Ryazanova, R.A., Druzhinina, V.A. & Nevstrueva, V.V. (1972) Experimental data for substantiating the maximum permissible concentration of zineb in the air of working premises. Gig. i Sanit., 50, 42-45

Seidler, H., Härtig, M., Schnaak, W. & Engst, R. (1970) Untersuchungen über den Metabolismus einiger Insektizide und Fungizide in der Ratte. II. Verteilung und Abbau von ^{14}C-markiertem Maneb. Die Nahrung, 14, 363-373

Sen, N.P., Donaldson, B.A. & Charbonneau, C. (1974) Formation of nitroso-dimethylamine from the interaction of certain pesticides and nitrite. In: Bogovski, P. & Walker, E.A., eds, N-Nitroso Compounds in the Environment, Lyon, IARC (IARC Scientific Publications No. 9), pp. 75-79

Stecher, P.G., ed. (1968) The Merck Index, 8th ed., Rahway, NJ, Merck & Co.

Strömme, J.H. (1965) Metabolism of disulfiram and diethyldithiocarbamate in rats with demonstration of an in vivo ethanol-induced inhibition of the glucuronic acid conjugation of the thiol. Biochem. Pharmacol., 14, 393-410

Sullivan, L.J., Eldridge, J.M., Knaak, J.B. & Tallant, M.J. (1972) 5,6-Di-hydro-5,6-dihydroxycarbaryl glucuronide as a significant metabolite of carbaryl in the rat. J. agric. Fd Chem., 20, 980-985

Tannenbaum, S.R., Sinskey, A.J., Weisman, M. & Bishop, W. (1974) Nitrite in human saliva. Its possible relationship to nitrosamine formation. J. nat. Cancer Inst., 53, 79-84

Truhaut, R., Fujita, M., Lich, N.P. & Chaigneau, M. (1973) Etude des trans-formations métaboliques du zinèbe (éthylène bisdithiocarbamate de zinc) chez le rat. C.R. Acad. Sci. (Paris), 276, 229-233

Ungerer, O., Eisenbrand, G. & Preussmann, R. (1974) Zur Reaktion von Nitrit mit Pestiziden. Bildung, chemische Eigenschaften und cancerogene Wirkung der N-Nitrosoverbindung des Herbizids N-Methyl-N'-(2-benzothiazolyl)-Harnstoff (Benzthiazuron). Z. Krebsforsch., 81, 217-224

Van Duuren, B.L., Goldschmidt, B.M., Katz, C. & Seidman, I. (1972) Dimethyl-carbamoyl chloride, a multipotential carcinogen. J. nat. Cancer Inst., 48, 1539-1541

Watts, R.R., Storherr, R.W. & Onley, J.H. (1974) Effects of cooking on ethylenebisdithiocarbamate degradation to ethylene thiourea. Bull. environm. Contam. Toxicol., 12, 224-226

Weisburger, E.K., Ulland, B.M., Schueler, R.L., Weisburger, J.H. & Harris, P.N. (1975) Carcinogenicity of three dose levels of 1,4-bis(4-fluorophenyl)-2-propynyl-N-cyclooctyl carbamate in male Sprague-Dawley and F344 rats. J. nat. Cancer Inst., 54, 975-979

WHO (1974) 1973 Evaluations of some pesticide residues in food. Wld Hlth Org. Pest. Res. Ser., No. 3, pp. 141-176

THE MONOGRAPHS

CARBARYL

1. Chemical and Physical Data

1.1 Synonyms and trade names

Chem. Abstr. Reg. Serial No.: 63-25-2

Chem. Abstr. Name: Methylcarbamate 1-naphthalenol

Methylcarbamate 1-naphthol; methylcarbamic acid, 1-naphthyl ester;
N-methylcarbamic acid, 1-naphthyl ester; *N*-methyl-1-naphthyl carbamate;
N-methyl-α-naphthylcarbamate; *N*-methyl-α-naphthylurethan; 1-naphthol
N-methylcarbamate; 1-naphthyl methylcarbamate; 1-naphthyl *N*-methyl
carbamate; α-naphthyl-*N*-methylcarbamate

Arylam; Atoxan; Caprolin; Carbatox; Carbatox-60; Carbatox 75;
Carpolin; Compound 7744; Denapon; Dicarbam; Gamonil; Germain's;
Hexavin; Karbaspray; Karbatox; Karbosep; NAC; Panam; Ravyon;
Septene; Sevimol; Sevin; Tricarnam; UC 7744; Union Carbide 7,744

1.2 Chemical formula and molecular weight

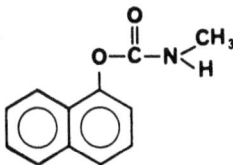

$C_{12}H_{11}NO_2$ Mol. wt: 201.2

1.3 Chemical and physical properties of the substance

From Stecher (1968), unless otherwise specified

(a) Description: Crystals

(b) Melting-point: 145°C

(c) Solubility: Slightly soluble in water at 25°C; soluble in
acetone, cyclohexanone, dimethylformamide and isophorone

(d) Volatility: Vapour pressure is <0.005 mm at 26°C (Frear, 1963).

(e) Stability: Stable to light and heat up to 70°C (Frear, 1963); hydrolysed rapidly by alkalis

1.4 Technical products and impurities

Carbaryl is available in the US and Japan as a technical grade product containing at least 99% of the compound. A partially formulated, finely ground grade of 95% purity is available in the US for use in the manufacture of more dilute, solid formulations. Formulations of carbaryl for various uses include wettable powders, dusts, granular products, suspensions, emulsifiable concentrate solutions and bait formulations (von Rumker *et al.*, 1974).

2. Production, Use, Occurrence and Analysis

For important background information on this section, see preamble, p. 15.

2.1 Production and use

Carbaryl can be synthesized by reacting phosgene with l-naphthol, followed by reaction with methylamine (Lambrech, 1959). Both this method and the reaction of l-naphthol with methyl isocyanate can be used for its commercial production (von Rumker *et al.*, 1974); the latter is believed to be used currently in the US.

Commercial production of carbaryl in the US was first reported in 1960 (US Tariff Commission, 1961). In 1972, US production was reported to be 24 million kg, of which 12.7 million kg were exported (von Rumker *et al.*, 1974).

It is estimated that about 5-10 million kg carbaryl are produced in the Federal Republic of Germany annually. Technical grade carbaryl is not produced in Japan; annual imports during the period 1970-74 averaged 1.04 million kg, with a peak of 1.17 million kg in 1971. About 200 thousand kg carbaryl, presumably in formulated form, were exported from Japan in 1974 (Japanese Ministry of Agriculture and Forestry, 1975).

The major use for carbaryl is as a broad spectrum insecticide, but it is also registered in the US as an acaricide and molluscicide. It is used for the control of insects which attack fruits, vegetables, cotton, tobacco, corn, rice, sugar beets, animals and livestock, and ornamental trees and shrubs (US Environmental Protection Agency, 1972). About 0.6 million kg are used annually in Italy.

According to the US Occupational Safety and Health Administration health standards for air contaminants, an employee's exposure to carbaryl should not exceed a time-weighted average of 5 mg/m^3 in the workplace air during any eight-hour work shift (US Code of Federal Regulations, 1975). In the USSR, the maximum allowable concentration in working atmospheres is 1 mg/m^3 (Winell, 1975).

Residue tolerances on raw agricultural commodities have been established in the US (US Code of Federal Regulations, 1974). Recommended tolerances were also established at the Joint Meeting of the FAO Working Party of Experts on Pesticide Residues and by the WHO Expert Committee on Pesticide Residues in December 1973; at the same time these two groups established an acceptable daily intake of carbaryl for man of 0-0.01 mg/kg bw (WHO, 1974).

2.2 Occurrence

Carbaryl is not known to occur as a natural product.

In a continuing programme involving the monitoring of pesticide residues in food, the US Department of Health, Education and Welfare found an increasing level of carbaryl in food samples collected at retail outlets during the period 1968-71. Between June 1970 and April 1971, carbaryl was found in leafy, legume and root vegetables, and in garden and tree fruits. Of 270 composite food samples examined, carbaryl was found in 20; in 15 of these it was found only at trace levels (Manske & Corneliussen, 1974).

2.3 Analysis

The Association of Official Analytical Chemists (Horwitz, 1975) has issued standard methods for carbaryl analysis, including a colorimetric method in which *para*-nitrobenzenediazonium fluoborate is used as a colour reagent; the developed colour is read spectrophotometrically. A modification of this method has been described (Kurtz & Studholme, 1974). McDermott (1973, 1975) reported modifications to the extraction technique of an earlier AOAC method. A procedure involving extraction and hydrolysis followed by the addition of *ortho*-toluidine had a sensitivity of 0.1-1 µg/ 20 mg sample (Rangaswamy & Majumder, 1974).

Column chromatography has been used to separate carbamates, such as carbaryl, which are then identified by thin-layer chromatography (Lichtenberg, 1975) or by gas chromatography and electron-capture detection after derivatization (Sherma & Shafik, 1975). The sensitivity of the latter method allowed detection of 40-2000 ng.

Weyer (1974) developed a gas-liquid chromatographic method for determining carbaryl directly in formulations. A high-pressure liquid chromatographic method for determining carbaryl at ambient temperatures had a reported sensitivity of greater than 7 ng (Colvin *et al.*, 1974). By the use of direct gas chromatography coupled with an alkali flame detector, recoveries of 90-100% over a range of 4-2000 ng have been reported (Lorah & Hemphill, 1974).

Thin-layer chromatography has been used to determine the carbaryl content of biological samples: after extraction and hydrolysis, the coloured compounds from the resulting l-naphthol were applied to thin-layer plates; as little as 0.01 µg carbaryl could be detected (Malinin, 1974).

A water monitoring system for cholinesterase inhibitors, including, but not specific for, carbaryl, uses an electrochemical cell which measures changes in the activity of immobilized enzymes (Goodson & Jacobs, 1972).

3. Biological Data Relevant to the Evaluation of Carcinogenic Risk to Man

3.1 Carcinogenicity and related studies in animals

(a) Oral administration

Mouse: Groups of 18 male and 18 female (C57BL/6xC3H/Anf)F_1 mice and 18 male and 18 female (C57BL/6xAKR)F_1 mice received commercial carbaryl (m.p. 141-142°C) according to the following schedule: 4.64 mg/kg bw in gelatine at 7 days of age by stomach tube and the same amount (not adjusted

40

for increasing body weight) daily up to 4 weeks of age; subsequently, the mice were given 14 mg carbaryl per kg of diet. The dose was the maximum tolerated dose for infant and young mice but not necessarily so for adults. The experiment was terminated when the animals were about 78 weeks of age, at which time 16, 18, 17 and 18 mice in the four groups, respectively, were still alive. Tumour incidences were compared with those observed among 79-90 necropsied mice of each sex and strain, which either had been untreated or had received gelatine only: the incidences were not significantly greater (P>0.05) for any tumour type in any sex-strain subgroup or in the combined sexes of either strain (Innes *et al*., 1969; NTIS, 1968).

Rat: Of 60 random-bred rats given 30 mg/kg bw commercial carbaryl (97.7% pure) in water by stomach tube daily for up to 22 months, 12 survivors were examined: 3 had fibrosarcomas, and 1 had an osteosarcoma. One fibro-sarcoma occurred among 46 untreated controls which survived 22 months (Andrianova & Alekseev, 1970) [P<0.01].

Groups of 20 male and 20 female CF-N rats were fed diets containing 0 (control), 0.005 (2 mg/kg bw/day), 0.01 (4 mg/kg bw/day), 0.02 (8 mg/kg bw/day) or 0.04% (16 mg/kg bw/day) carbaryl; survivors were killed after 732-736 days. The mean ages at death for both sexes at the 0.04 and 0.02% levels were 656 and 630 days, and that for controls, 585 days. The incidence of tumours in carbaryl-treated rats was no different from that in controls; tumour types were not reported (Carpenter *et al*., 1961).

(b) Subcutaneous administration

Mouse: Groups of 18 male and 18 female (C57BL/6xC3H/Anf)F_1 mice and 18 male and 18 female (C57BL/6xAKR)F_1 mice were given single s.c. injections of 100 mg/kg bw commercial carbaryl (m.p. 141-142°C) in dimethyl sulphoxide on the 28th day of life and were observed until they were about 78 weeks of age, at which time 15, 18, 18 and 17 mice in the four groups, respectively, were still alive. Tumour incidences were compared with those in groups of 141, 154, 161 and 157 untreated or vehicle-injected controls that were necropsied. Incidences were not significantly increased (P>0.05) for any tumour type in any sex-strain subgroup or in the combined sexes of either strain (NTIS, 1968) [The Working Group noted that a negative result obtained after a single s.c. injection may not be an adequate basis for discounting carcinogenicity].

Groups of 30 3-month old male A/Jax or C3H mice were given s.c. injections weekly over 5 months of 10 mg/animal carbaryl in 0.2 ml agar suspension, the agar suspension alone or left untreated. The number of lung tumours seen at 8 months of age was no greater in treated than in control mice (Carpenter *et al.*, 1961).

Rat: Of 48 random-bred rats given a s.c. implant of 20 mg/kg commercial carbaryl (97.7% pure) in a 250 mg paraffin pellet, 10 survived 22 months; 2 had subcutaneous sarcomas at the site of implantation. One fibrosarcoma occurred among 46 controls, which did not receive paraffin pellets and were still alive at 22 months (Andrianova & Alekseev, 1970) [P>0.05].

(c) Intraperitoneal administration

Mouse: Of 16 7-9-week old male A/He mice given 12 i.p. injections of carbaryl (purity not given) in tricaprylin over 4 weeks (total dose, 6 mg/animal), 6 out of 15 mice still alive 20 weeks after the end of the treatment and then killed developed lung tumours. Of tricaprylin-injected controls, 7/28 animals developed a total of 8 lung tumours; 2/31 untreated controls had 1 lung tumour each (Shimkin *et al.*, 1969) [P>0.05].

3.2 Other relevant biological data

(a) Experimental systems

The oral LD_{50} for carbaryl in mice is 438 mg/kg bw (Rybakova, 1966). Oral LD_{50}'s in rats, female rats and rabbits are 510, 610 and 710 mg/kg bw, respectively (Carpenter *et al.*, 1961).

No toxic effects were seen in rats administered up to 200 mg carbaryl per kg of diet for 2 years. With higher dietary levels (1500 and 2250 mg/kg of diet), diffuse, cloudy swelling of the kidney tubules was seen after 96 days (Carpenter *et al.*, 1961).

Neurotoxicological effects of carbaryl (200 mg/kg of diet/day for 50 days) have been shown in Wistar rats (i) to affect learning (after 25 days) and performance (after 15 days), (ii) to affect electroencephalographic patterns under resting and light-stimulated conditions, and (iii) to inhibit

42

acetylcholinesterase activity in the erythrocytes and in various parts of
the brain. Mild but permanent and increasing functional deviations of the
central nervous system were found (Dési et al., 1974). Marked functional
and structural changes of the pituitary gland with impairment of thyroid
and gonadal function have been found in rats administered 7, 14 or 70 mg
carbaryl/kg bw/day for up to 12 months (Shtenberg & Rybakova, 1968).

Of an oral dose of [1-naphthyl-1-^{14}C]-N-methylcarbamate given to rats,
53% and 82% were absorbed after 20 min and 1 hour, respectively (Casper
et al., 1973). Carbaryl is absorbed very rapidly from the lung, 2.5 times
faster than from the small intestine (Hwang & Schanker, 1974).

The distribution of carbaryl, ^{14}C-labelled at various positions, was
investigated by Knaak et al. (1965) in rats and guinea-pigs and by
Krishna & Casida (1966) in rats. The relatively longer retention of
^{14}C after oral administration of [N-methyl-^{14}C]-carbaryl may indicate
methylcarbamoylation of proteins in vivo after carbaryl hydrolysis
(Strother, 1972); 25% of the carbamate ester was hydrolysed (Kuhr &
Dorough, 1976), and the 1-naphthol produced was rapidly excreted.
Excretions of carbaryl after enteral and parenteral administrations were
similar.

Carbaryl (1) (Scheme 1) was metabolized by rat liver microsomes to
1-naphthyl-N-hydroxymethylcarbamate (2), 4-hydroxy-1-naphthyl-N-methyl-
carbamate (3), 5-hydroxy-1-naphthyl-N-methylcarbamate (4) and 5,6-dihydroxy-
5,6-dihydro-1-naphthyl-N-methylcarbamate (5) (Dorough & Casida, 1964;
Dorough et al., 1963; Hassan et al., 1966; Kuhr & Dorough, 1976). Human
and rat liver homogenates produced equal amounts (3.4%) of the 4- and 5-hydroxy
derivatives (3) and (4) when incubated with carbaryl, although much of the
parent compound (72 and 58%, respectively) was recovered unchanged; more
1-naphthyl-N-hydroxymethylcarbamate was formed by rat liver (4%) than by
human liver (<1%) (Matsumura & Ward, 1966; Strother, 1970, 1972). Hydrolytic
products included 1-naphthol (6) (Dorough & Casida, 1964).

Epoxidation is implicit from the identification of compounds (3), (4)
and (5) (Bend et al., 1971). Among the metabolites found in the urine of
treated rats were the mercapturic acids S-(4-hydroxy-1-naphthyl)cysteine (7)
and S-(5-hydroxy-1-naphthyl)cysteine (9) (Bend et al., 1971) and the

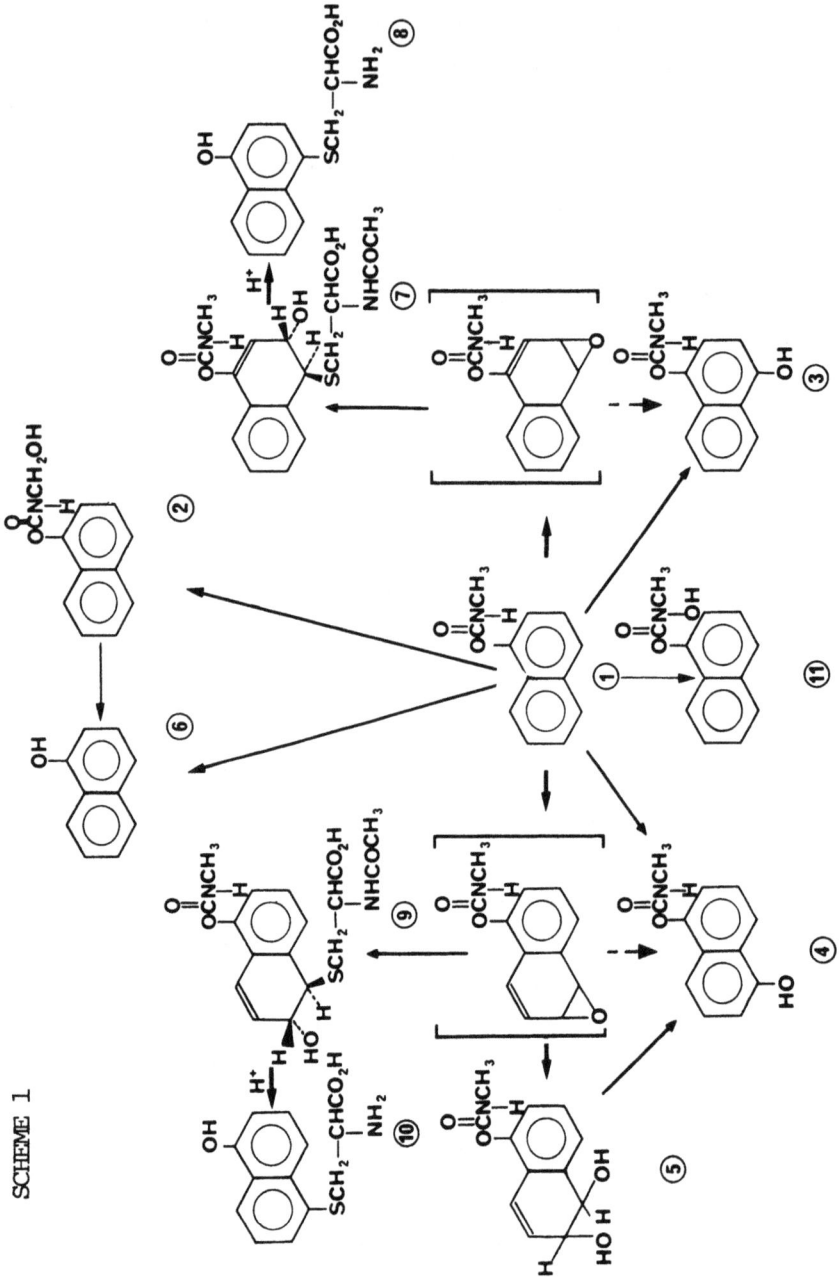

SCHEME 1

44

glucuronide of (5) (Sullivan *et al.*, 1972). Another metabolite, 1-naphthyl-
N-hydroxy-*N*-methylcarbamate (11), has been identified in rat-liver preparations
incubated with carbaryl (Locke, 1972). Compound (5) has been identified
as a metabolite in bovine milk (Baron *et al.*, 1969), and (1), (2), (3) and
(6) have been found in smaller quantities (Camp *et al.*, 1963; Dorough,
1967; Whitehurst *et al.*, 1963).

Cress & Strother (1974) have shown that carbaryl induces microsomal
hepatic mixed-function oxidase in mice.

Ingestion of carbaryl by beagle dogs throughout gestation caused teratogenic effects at all but the lowest dose level (3.125 mg/kg bw/day).
Embryopathies in 21 out of a total of 181 pups were characterized by
abdominal-thoracic fissures with varying degrees of brachygnathia, ecaudate
pups, failure of skeletal formation and superfluous phalanges (Smalley *et
al.*, 1968). Carbaryl was teratogenic in guinea-pigs when administered
during organogenesis at 300 mg/kg bw/day, but not in hamsters (at 250 mg/kg
bw) or in rabbits (at 200 mg/kg bw) (Robens, 1969). No effects on reproduction occurred in rats given 200 mg/kg bw daily in the diet, but reduced
fertility was seen in those given 100 mg/kg bw daily intragastrically
(Weil *et al.*, 1972).

The reaction of carbaryl with nitrous acid leads to formation of *N*-nitro-
socarbaryl (Elespuru & Lijinsky, 1973). This proceeds less readily at lower
concentrations (Eisenbrand *et al.*, 1975), but formation of *N*-nitrosocarbaryl in
the stomach could be expected. *N*-Nitrosocarbaryl, without metabolic activation,
is a potent bacterial mutagen (Elespuru *et al.*, 1974; Lijinsky & Elespuru,
1976) and is mutagenic in yeast (Siebert & Eisenbrand, 1974). It is carcinogenic in rats after its oral administration (Eisenbrand *et al.*, 1976;
Lijinsky & Taylor, 1976) and after single subcutaneous injections (Eisenbrand
et al., 1975). *N*-Nitrosocarbaryl interacts with human DNA *in vitro*, producing
alkali-sensitive bonds (Regan *et al.*, 1976). These authors also found that,
in contrast to its *N*-nitroso derivative, [methyl-^{14}C]-carbaryl did not bind
to the DNA of human skin cells from normal subjects or from those with
xeroderma pigmentosum.

Carbaryl inhibits spindle fibre formation in plants (Amer, 1965; Amer & Farah, 1968; Wuu & Grant, 1966). Inhibition of mitosis and spindle fibre formation has also been reported in cultured human embryonic fibroblasts after treatment with 20-80 µg/ml of a technical product containing 84% carbaryl (Vasilos *et al.*, 1972).

No reverse mutations were observed in a spot test on *Escherichia coli* (Ashwood-Smith *et al.*, 1972), and no mitotic gene conversion was seen in *Saccharomyces cerevisiae* (Siebert & Eisenbrand, 1974); metabolic activation systems were not used in these tests. In the presence of an Aroclor-induced, rat-liver microsomal preparation carbaryl was not mutagenic to TA100, TA98, TA1535 or TA1537 strains of *Salmonella typhimurium* (McCann *et al.*, 1975).

Carbaryl (85% purity) caused an increased number of recessive lethals in *Drosophila melanogaster* (Brzeskij & Vaskov, 1971). No increase of dominant lethals in mice was recorded after five oral treatments with 50 or 1000 mg/kg (Epstein *et al.*, 1972). In a dominant lethal test in male rats fed up to 200 mg/kg carbaryl per day in the diet or up to 100 mg/kg per day by oral intubation until 224 days of age, no increase in dominant lethality could be established (Weil *et al.*, 1973) [The data is difficult to evaluate since results are given as the percentage of pregnant females with one or more foetal deaths, and the actual frequency of live or dead foetuses is not given].

(b) Man

Workers engaged in the production, collection and bagging of carbaryl were exposed by inhalation to 0.23-31 mg dust/m^3; they excreted up to 80 mg 1-naphthol/day but showed only slight depression of blood acetylcholinesterase activity (Best & Murray, 1962).

A large proportion of carbaryl applied to the forearms of human volunteers was absorbed, and 74% of the dose was excreted in the urine (Feldmann & Maibach, 1974).

The urinary metabolites in humans who ingested carbaryl included the glucuronides of (3) (Scheme 1) and (6) (Knaak *et al.*, 1968). The metabolic activity of human organ cultures *in vitro* was in the order liver>lungs>

kidneys>placenta>vaginal mucosa>uterus and uterine leiomyoma (Chin *et al.*, 1974). Human liver microsomal preparations gave the 4- and 5-hydroxy derivatives (3) and (4) when incubated with carbaryl, although 72% of the parent compound was recovered unchanged (Strother, 1972).

Human volunteers who ingested 0.12 mg/kg bw carbaryl/day for 6 weeks showed a decrease in the ratio of amino acid:creatinine nitrogen in the urine (Wills *et al.*, 1968).

3.3 Case reports and epidemiological studies

No data were available to the Working Group.

4. Comments on Data Reported and Evaluation

4.1 Animal data

In one study in rats with relatively low survival rates, carbaryl produced sarcomas following its oral but not after its subcutaneous administration. In one study in mice by oral administration, no carcinogenic effect was observed. The available data not not allow an evaluation of the carcinogenicity of carbaryl to be made.

Carbaryl can react with nitrite under mildly acid conditions, simulating those in the human stomach, to give rise to N-nitrosocarbaryl, which has been shown to be carcinogenic in rats (see also 'General Remarks on Carbamates, Thiocarbamates and Carbazides', pp. 25-27).

4.2 Human data

No case reports or epidemiological studies were available to the Working Group.

5. References

Amer, S.M. (1965) Cytological effects of pesticides. I. Mitotic effects of *N*-methyl-1-naphthyl carbamate 'Sevin'. Cytologia, 30, 175-181

Amer, S.M. & Farah, O.R. (1968) Cytological effects of pesticides. III. Meiotic effects of *N*-methyl-1-naphthyl carbamate 'Sevin'. Cytologia, 33, 337-344

Andrianova, M.M. & Alekseev, I.V. (1970) On the carcinogenic properties of the pesticides sevine, maneb, ciram and cineb. Vop. Pitan., 29, 71-74

Ashwood-Smith, M.J., Trevino, J. & Ring, R. (1972) Mutagenicity of dichlorvos. Nature (Lond.), 240, 418-420

Baron, R.L., Sphon, J.A., Chen, J.T., Lustig, E., Doherty, J.D., Hansen, E.A. & Kolbye, S.M. (1969) Confirmatory isolation and identification of a metabolite of carbaryl in urine and milk. J. agric. Fd Chem., 17, 883-887

Bend, J.R., Holder, G.M., Protos, E. & Ryan, A.J. (1971) Water-soluble metabolites of carbaryl (1-naphthyl *N*-methylcarbamate) in mouse-liver preparations and in the rat. Austr. J. biol. Sci., 24, 535-546

Best, E.M., Jr & Murray, B.L. (1962) Observations on workers exposed to sevin insecticide: a preliminary report. J. occup. Med., 4, 507-517

Brzeskij, V.V. & Vaskov, V.I. (1971) Mutationsuntersuchungen und Fertilitätsberechnung bei *Drosophila melanogaster* unter Carbarylwirkung. Angew. Parasitol., 13, 23-28

Camp, H.B., Buttram, J.R., Hays, K.L. & Arthur, B.W. (1963) Sevin residues in milk from dairy cows following dermal applications. J. econ. Entomol., 56, 402-404

Carpenter, C.P., Weil, C.S., Palm, P.E., Woodside, M.W., Nair, J.H., III & Smyth, H.F., Jr (1961) Mammalian toxicity of 1-naphthyl-*N*-methyl-carbamate (sevin insecticide). J. agric. Fd Chem., 9, 30-39

Casper, H.H., Pekas, J.C. & Dinusson, W.E. (1973) Gastric absorption of a pesticide (1-naphthyl *N*-methylcarbamate) in the fasted rat. Pest. Biochem. Physiol., 2, 391-396

Chin, B.H., Eldridge, J.M. & Sullivan, L.J. (1974) Metabolism of carbaryl by selected human tissues using an organ-maintenance technique. Clin. Toxicol., 7, 37-56

Colvin, B.M., Engdahl, B.S. & Hanks, A.R. (1974) Determination of carbaryl in pesticide formulations and fertilizers by high-pressure liquid chromatography. J. Ass. off. analyt. Chem., 57, 648-652

Cress, C.R. & Strother, A. (1974) Effects on drug metabolism of carbaryl and 1-naphthol in the mouse. Life Sci., 14, 861-872

Dési, I., Gönczi, L., Simon, G., Farkas, I. & Kneffel, Z. (1974) Neurotoxicological studies of two carbamate pesticides in subacute animal experiments. Toxicol. appl. Pharmacol., 27, 465-476

Dorough, H.W. (1967) Carbaryl-C^{14} metabolism in a lactating cow. J. agric. Fd Chem., 15, 261-266

Dorough, H.W. & Casida, J.E. (1964) Nature of certain carbamate metabolites of the insecticide sevin. J. agric. Fd Chem., 12, 294-304

Dorough, H.W., Leeling, N.C. & Casida, J.E. (1963) Non-hydrolytic pathway in metabolism of N-methylcarbamate insecticides. Science, 140, 170-171

Eisenbrand, G., Ungerer, O. & Preussmann, R. (1975) The reaction of nitrite with pesticides. II. Formation, chemical properties and carcinogenic activity of the N-nitroso derivative of N-methyl-1-naphthyl carbamate (carbaryl). Fd Cosmet. Toxicol., 13, 365-367

Eisenbrand, G., Schmähl, D. & Preussmann, R. (1976) Carcinogenicity in rats of high oral doses of N-nitrosocarbaryl, a nitrosated pesticide. Cancer Lett., 1, 281-284

Elespuru, R.K. & Lijinsky, W. (1973) The formation of carcinogenic nitroso compounds from nitrite and some types of agricultural chemicals. Fd Cosmet. Toxicol., 11, 807-817

Elespuru, R.K., Lijinsky, W. & Setlow, J.K. (1974) Nitrosocarbaryl as a potent mutagen of environmental significance. Nature (Lond.), 247, 386-387

Epstein, S.S., Arnold, E., Andrea, J., Bass, W. & Bishop, Y. (1972) Detection of chemical mutagens by the dominant lethal assay in the mouse. Toxicol. appl. Pharmacol., 23, 288-325

Feldmann, R.J. & Maibach, H.I. (1974) Percutaneous penetration of some pesticides and herbicides in man. Toxicol. appl. Pharmacol., 28, 126-132

Frear, D.E.H., ed. (1963) Pesticide Index, State College, Pennsylvania, College Science Publishers, p. 47

Goodson, L.H. & Jacobs, W.B. (1972) Rapid Detection System for Organophosphates and Carbamate Insecticides in Water, EPA-R2-72-010, Washington DC, US Environmental Protection Agency

Hassan, A., Zayed, S.M.A.D. & Abdel-Hamid, F.M. (1966) Metabolism of carbamate drugs. I. Metabolism of 1-naphthyl-N-methyl carbamate (sevin) in the rat. Biochem. Pharmacol., 15, 2045-2055

Horwitz, W., ed. (1975) Official Methods of Analysis, 12th ed., Washington DC, Association of Official Analytical Chemists, pp. 537-539

Hwang, S.W. & Schanker, L.S. (1974) Absorption of carbaryl from the lung and small intestine of the rat. Environm. Res., 7, 206-211

Innes, J.R.M., Ulland, B.M., Valerio, M.G., Petrucelli, L., Fishbein, L., Hart, E.R., Pallotta, A.J., Bates, R.R., Falk, H.L., Gart, J.J., Klein, M., Mitchell, I. & Peters, J. (1969) Bioassay of pesticides and industrial chemicals for tumorigenicity in mice: a preliminary note. J. nat. Cancer Inst., 42, 1101-1114

Japanese Ministry of Agriculture and Forestry (1975) Noyaku Yoran (Agricultural Chemicals Annual), 1975, Division of Plant Disease Prevention, Tokyo, Takeo Endo, pp. 85, 93, 224, 225

Knaak, J.B., Tallant, M.J., Bartley, W.J. & Sullivan, L.J. (1965) The metabolism of carbaryl in the rat, guinea pig and man. J. agric. Fd Chem., 13, 537-543

Knaak, J.B., Tallant, M.J., Kozbelt, S.J. & Sullivan, L.J. (1968) The metabolism of carbaryl in man, monkey, pig and sheep. J. agric. Fd Chem., 16, 465-470

Krishna, J.G. & Casida, J.E. (1966) Fate in rats of the radiocarbon from ten variously labelled methyl- and dimethyl-carbamate-^{14}C insecticide chemicals and their hydrolysis products. J. agric. Fd Chem., 14, 98-105

Kuhr, R.J. & Dorough H.W. (1976) Carbamate Insecticides: Chemistry, Biochemistry and Toxicology, Cleveland, Ohio, Chemical Rubber Co., p. 109

Kurtz, D.A. & Studholme, C.R. (1974) Recovery of trichlorfon (Dylox ®) and carbaryl (Sevin ®) in songbirds following spraying of forest for gypsy moth. Bull. environm. Contam. Toxicol., 11, 78-84

Lambrech, J.A. (1959) α-Naphthol bicyclic aryl esters of N-substituted carbamic acids, US Patent 2,903,478, September 8, to Union Carbide

Lichtenberg, J.J. (1975) Methods for the determination of specific organic pollutants in water and waste water. Inst. Electrical Electronics Engineers Trans. Nuclear Sci., NS-22, 874-891

Lijinsky, W. & Elespuru, R.K. (1976) Mutagenicity and carcinogenicity of N-nitroso derivatives of carbamate insecticides. In: Rosenfeld, C. & Davis, W., eds, Environmental Pollution and Carcinogenic Risks, Lyon, IARC (IARC Scientific Publications No. 13) (in press)

Lijinsky, W. & Taylor, H.W. (1976) Carcinogenesis in Sprague-Dawley rats by N-nitroso-N-alkylcarbamate esters. Cancer Lett., 1, 275-279

Locke, R.K. (1972) Thin-layer chromatography of 1-naphthyl *N*-hydroxy-*N*-methylcarbamate and its application in two *in vitro* studies involving carbaryl. J. agric. Fd Chem., 20, 1078-1080

Lorah, E.J. & Hemphill, D.D. (1974) Direct chromatography of some *N*-methyl-carbamate pesticides. J. Ass. off. analyt. Chem., 57, 570-575

Malinin, O.A. (1974) Determination of sevin in biological specimens. Veterinariya (Moscow), 2, 104-105

Manske, D.D. & Corneliussen, P.E. (1974) Pesticide residues in total diet samples. VII. Pest. Monit. J., 8, 110-114

Matsumura, F. & Ward, C.T. (1966) Degradation of insecticides by the human and the rat liver. Arch. environm. Hlth, 13, 257-261

McCann, J., Choi, E., Yamasaki, E. & Ames, B.N. (1975) Detection of carcinogens as mutagens in the *Salmonella*/microsome test: assay of 300 chemicals. Proc. nat. Acad. Sci. (Wash.), 72, 5135-5139

McDermott, W.H. (1973) Infrared analysis of carbaryl insecticide: modification of the extraction procedure to accommodate liquid suspension formulations. J. Ass. off. analyt. Chem., 56, 576-578

McDermott, W.H. (1975) Carbaryl insecticide: extraction from dust and powder formulations. J. Ass. off. analyt. Chem., 58, 28-32

NTIS (National Technical Information Service) (1968) Evaluation of Carcinogenic, Teratogenic and Mutagenic Activities of Selected Pesticides and Industrial Chemicals, Vol. 1, Carcinogenic Study, Washington DC, US Department of Commerce

Rangaswamy, J.R. & Majumder, S.K. (1974) Colorimetric method for estimation of carbaryl and its residues on grains. J. Ass. off. analyt. Chem., 57, 592-594

Regan, J.D., Setlow, R.B., Francis, A.A. & Lijinsky, W. (1976) Nitrosocarbaryl: its effect on human DNA. Mutation Res., 38, 293-302

Robens, J.F. (1969) Teratologic studies of carbaryl, diazinon, norea, disulfiram and thiram in small laboratory animals. Toxicol. appl. Pharmacol., 15, 152-163

von Rumker, R., Lawless, E.W. & Meiners, A.F. (1974) Production, Distribution, Use, and Environmental Impact Potential of Selected Pesticides, Washington DC, US Environmental Protection Agency, pp. 133-136

Rybakova, M.N. (1966) On the toxic effect of sevine on animals. Gig. i Sanit., 31, 42-47

Sherma, J. & Shafik, T.M. (1975) A multiclass, multiresidue analytical method for determining pesticide residues in air. Arch. environm. Contam. Toxicol., 3, 55-71

Shimkin, M.B., Wieder, R., McDonough, M., Fishbein, L. & Swern, D. (1969) Lung tumor response in strain A mice as a quantitative bioassay of carcinogenic activity of some carbamates and aziridines. Cancer Res., 29, 2184-2190

Shtenberg, A.I. & Rybakova, M.N. (1968) Effect of carbaryl on the neuro-endocrine system of rats. Fd Cosmet. Toxicol., 6, 461-467

Siebert, D. & Eisenbrand, G. (1974) Induction of mitotic gene conversion in *Saccharomyces cerevisiae* by *N*-nitrosated pesticides. Mutation Res., 22, 121-126

Smalley, H.E., Curtis, J.M. & Earl, F.L. (1968) Teratogenic action of carbaryl in beagle dogs. Toxicol. appl. Pharmacol., 13, 392-403

Stecher, P.G., ed. (1968) The Merck Index, 8th ed., Rahway, NJ, Merck & Co., p. 104

Strother, A. (1970) Comparative metabolism of selected *N*-methylcarbamates by human and rat liver fractions. Biochem. Pharmacol., 19, 2525-2529

Strother, A. (1972) *In vitro* metabolism of methylcarbamate insecticides by human and rat liver fraction. Toxicol. appl. Pharmacol., 21, 112-129

Sullivan, L.J., Eldridge, J.M., Knaak, J.B. & Tallant, M.J. (1972) 5,6-Dihydro-5,6-dihydroxycarbaryl glucuronide as a significant metabolite of carbaryl in the rat. J. agric. Fd Chem., 20, 980-985

US Code of Federal Regulations (1974) Protection of Environment, Title 40, part. 180.169, Washington DC, US Government Printing Office, p. 262

US Code of Federal Regulations (1975) Air Contaminants, Title 29, part. 1910.1000, Washington DC, US Government Printing Office, pp. 59-60

US Environmental Protection Agency (1972) EPA Compendium of Registered Pesticides, Vol. III, Insecticides, Acaricides, Molluscicides and Antifouling Compounds, Washington DC, US Government Printing Office, p. III-C-7

US Tariff Commission (1961) Synthetic Organic Chemicals, US Production and Sales, 1960, TC Publication 34, Washington DC, US Government Printing Office, p. 161

Vasilos, A.F., Dmitrienko, V.D. & Shroit, I.G. (1972) Colchicine-like action of sevine on human embryonic fibroblasts *in vitro*. Byull. eksp. biol. Med., 73, 91-93

Weil, C.S., Woodside, M.D., Carpenter, C.P. & Smyth, H.F., Jr (1972) Current status of tests of carbaryl for reproductive and teratogenic effect. Toxicol. appl. Pharmacol., 21, 390-404

Weil, C.S., Woodside, M.D., Bernard, J.B., Condra, N.I., King, J.M. & Carpenter, C.P. (1973) Comparative effect of carbaryl on rat reproduction and guinea pig teratology when fed either in the diet or by stomach intubation. Toxicol. appl. Pharmacol., 26, 621-638

Weyer, L.G. (1974) Gas-liquid chromatographic method for the analysis of carbaryl insecticide formulations. J. Ass. off. analyt. Chem., 57, 778-780

Whitehurst, W.E., Bishop, E.T., Critchfield, F.E., Gyrisco, G.G., Huddleston, E.W., Arnold, H. & Lisk, D.J. (1963) The metabolism of sevin in dairy cows. J. agric. Fd Chem., 11, 167-169

WHO (1974) 1973 Evaluations of some pesticide residues in food. Wld Hlth Org. Pest. Res. Ser., No. 3, pp. 141-176

Wills, J.H., Jameson, E. & Coulston, F. (1968) Effects of oral doses of carbaryl on man. Clin. Toxicol., 1, 265-271

Winell, M.A. (1975) An international comparison of hygienic standards for chemicals in the work environment. Ambio, 4, 34-36

Wuu, K.D. & Grant, W.F. (1966) Morphological and somatic chromosomal aberrations induced by pesticides in barley (*Hordeum vulgare*). Canad. J. Genet. Cytol., 8, 481-501

CHLOROPROPHAM

1. Chemical and Physical Data

1.1 Synonyms and trade names

Chem. Abstr. Reg. Serial No.: 101-21-3

Chem. Abstr. Name: (3-Chlorophenyl)carbamic acid, 1-methylethyl ester

Chlor-IPC; *meta*-chlorocarbanilic acid, isopropyl ester; chloro-ICP; chloro IPC; (3-chlorophenyl)carbamic acid, isopropyl ester; *N*-(3-chlorophenyl)carbamic acid, isopropyl ester; *N*-3-chlorophenyliso-propylcarbamate; CICP; CI-IPC; CIPC; isopropyl 3-chlorocarbanilate; isopropyl *meta*-chlorocarbanilate; isopropyl 3-chlorophenylcarbamate; isopropyl *N*-3-chlorophenyl carbamate; *O*-isopropyl *N*-(3-chlorophenyl)-carbamate

Chlor IFC; Chlor-IFK; Chlorpropham; Elbanil; Furloe; Liro CIPC; Metoxon; Nexoval; Prevenol; Prevenol 56; Preventol; Preventol 56; Sprout Nip; Spud-Nie; Taterpex; Triherbicide CIPC; Triherbide-CIPC; Y 3

1.2 Chemical formula and molecular weight

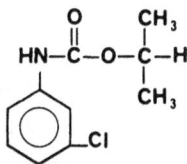

$C_{10}H_{12}ClNO_2$ Mol. wt: 213.7

1.3 Chemical and physical properties of the substance

From Stecher (1968), unless otherwise specified

(a) Description: Solid

(b) Boiling-point: $149^{\circ}C$ at 2 mm; $247^{\circ}C$ (decomposition) at 760 mm (Gard & Ferguson, 1964)

(c) Melting-point: $40.7-41.1^{\circ}C$

(d) <u>Refractive index</u>: n_D^{20} = 1.5395 (super-cooled) (Gard & Ferguson, 1964)

(e) <u>Solubility</u>: Slightly soluble in water (Gard & Ferguson, 1964); soluble in most oils and organic solvents

(f) <u>Volatility</u>: Vapour pressure is 10^{-5}-10^{-6} mm at 25°C (extrapolated) (Gard & Ferguson, 1964).

1.4 Technical products and impurities

The commercial product is a liquid (Stecher, 1968). Chloropropham is available in the US as an emulsifiable concentrate containing about 40% of the pure chemical and as granular formulations on an attapulgite clay base containing 10 or 20% by weight of the chemical (Weed Science Society of America, 1974).

In Japan, chloropropham is available as an emulsifiable concentrate containing 45.8% chloropropham and as a wettable powder containing 7.8% of the chemical (Japanese Ministry of Agriculture and Forestry, 1975).

2. Production, Use, Occurrence and Analysis

For important background information on this section, see preamble, p. 15.

2.1 Production and use

Chloropropham can be prepared either by the reaction of 3-chlorophenyl isocyanate with isopropyl alcohol or by the reaction of 3-chloroaniline with isopropyl chloroformate (Weed Science Society of America, 1974).

It has been produced commercially in the US since 1951 (US Tariff Commission, 1952), but only one US company now does so. The amount produced is estimated to have reached about 300 thousand kg in 1964 and to have decreased to a level of approximately 225 thousand kg in 1971.

There are reported to be two producers of chloropropham in the UK and one in The Netherlands (Berg, 1975). Annual production of chloropropham in Europe is estimated to be less than 1 million kg.

It has been produced in Japan since 1962 by one company, which produced 62 thousand kg in 1974. Imports in that year were 73 thousand kg (Japanese Ministry of Agriculture and Forestry, 1975).

The only known use of chloropropham is as a highly selective pre-emergence and early post-emergence herbicide. It is registered for use in the US on about 20 crops, including forage, vegetable, fruit and field crops. Residue tolerances in the US have been established in the range of 0.1-0.3 mg/kg for all crops except forage, for which tolerances are from 20-50 mg/kg (US Environmental Protection Agency, 1974). The quantity of chloropropham used on US agricultural crops in 1971 is estimated to have been approximately 200 thousand kg. Only 9 thousand kg, applied to 5 thousand acres of cropland, were used in the state of California in 1974 (California Department of Food & Agriculture, 1975).

In Japan, the following crops are treated with this chemical for weed control (listed in order of quantities of chloropropham used): vegetables (especially onions and potatoes), wheat, fruit, flowers and vegetables, turf, miscellaneous herbs and strawberries (Japanese Ministry of Agriculture and Forestry, 1975).

2.2 Occurrence

Chloropropham does not occur as a natural product. Residual amounts may occur on or in treated crops after harvesting.

2.3 Analysis

There are several reviews which include methods of analysis for chloropropham (Fishbein, 1975; Fishbein & Zielinski, 1967; Gard & Ferguson, 1964; Sherma, 1973; Zweig & Sherma, 1972).

Gas chromatography with electron capture detection of the brominated aniline, produced by a one-step hydrolysis and bromination, was used to determine chloropropham extracted from fruit and vegetables. The method is sensitive to about 0.02 mg/kg (Gutenmann & Lisk, 1964). Gas chromatography with electrolytic conductivity detection of chloropropham after alkylation has been used to determine chloropropham extracted from crops at a limit of detection of about 0.005 mg/kg (Lawrence & Laver, 1975). A method for systematic identification and determination of a number of pesticides, including chloropropham, using a combination of column, thin-layer and gas chromatography, has been described; 200 ng of chloropropham could readily be detected (Suzuki *et al.*, 1974). Both thin-layer chromatography and high-speed liquid chromatography have been used to separate and detect fluorescent derivatives of the amine produced by alkaline hydrolysis of a number of carbamate and urea herbicides. The thin-layer chromatographic method was applicable to the quantitative analysis of residues in selected crops at a detection limit of 0.05 mg/kg (Lawrence & Laver, 1974); 1-10 ng could be detected by high-speed liquid chromatography (Frei & Lawrence, 1973).

A colorimetric method which measures the 3-chloroaniline formed on alkaline hydrolysis of chloropropham has been used to determine residues in alfalfa. The method includes a clean-up technique which eliminates inter-fering plant materials and has a limit of detection of 0.02 mg/kg (Ercegovich & Witkonton, 1972). Basically the same colorimetric technique, with a different clean-up procedure, has been adapted to an automated system for the analysis of vegetables (Friestad, 1974) and soils (Burge & Gross, 1972), and has a detection limit of about 0.01 mg/kg.

3. Biological Data Relevant to the Evaluation of Carcinogenic Risk to Man

3.1 Carcinogenicity and related studies in animals

(a) Oral administration

Mouse: Groups of 18 male and 18 female (C57BL/6xC3H/Anf)F_1 mice and 18 male and 18 female (C57BL/6xAKR)F_1 mice received commercial chloro-propham (98.5% pure) according to the following schedule: 464 mg/kg bw in gelatine at 7 days of age by stomach tube and the same amount (not adjusted for increasing body weight) daily up to 4 weeks of age; subsequently, the mice were given 1112 mg chloropropham per kg of diet. The dose was the maximum tolerated dose for infant and young mice but not necessarily so for adults. The experiment was terminated when the animals were about 78 weeks of age, at which time 14, 18, 15 and 16 mice in the four groups, respectively, were still alive. Tumour incidences were compared with those observed among

79-90 necropsied mice of each sex and strain, which either had been untreated or had received gelatine only: the incidences were not significantly greater (P>0.05) for any tumour type in any sex-strain subgroup or in the combined sexes of either strain (Innes *et al.*, 1969; NTIS, 1968).

A group of 25 male and 25 female 7-week old Swiss mice was given 1000 mg chloropropham (m.p. 40-41°C; containing 30-40 mg/kg chloroaniline) per kg of diet for up to 116 weeks, when the survivors were killed. The average lifespans were 78 weeks in treated males and 84 weeks in treated females, compared with 75 weeks in 25 male and 25 female controls fed the standard diet; 36/47 treated mice had tumours, compared with 33/49 controls. Lung adenomas were observed in 15/47 treated mice, compared with 10/49 in controls (van Esch & Kroes, 1972).

Rat: In a 2-year study, 4 groups of 25 male and 25 female young albino rats were given 0, 200, 2000 or 20,000 mg chloropropham (purity not specified) per kg of diet; of the animals alive at 91 weeks, 4/9 female and 2/11 male controls had tumours in various organs, as did 2/10 and 1/11 animals in the group given 200 mg per kg of diet, 3/16 and 2/5 in the group given 2000 mg per kg of diet and 1/10 and 3/5 in the group given 20,000 mg per kg of diet (Larson *et al.*, 1960).

Hamster: A group of 23 male and 26 female hamsters was given 2000 mg chloropropham (m.p. 40-41°C; containing 30-40 mg/kg chloroaniline) per kg of diet for 33 months; a control group of 22 males and 27 females received the basal diet. After 2 years, 1 treated female, 1 control female, 13 treated males and 14 control males were alive. Bile-duct hyperplasia in the liver was observed in 19 treated animals and in 28 controls. Six tumours in different organs were seen in treated animals and 8 in controls (van Esch. & Kroes, 1972).

(b) Subcutaneous administration

Mouse: A group of 25 male and 25 female 7-week old Swiss mice was given 9 s.c. injections of 1000 mg/kg bw chloropropham (m.p. 40-41°C; containing 30-40 mg/kg chloroaniline) in 0.025 ml methylpyrrolidone at irregular intervals over 17 months. A control group of 25 mice was injected with methylpyrrolidone alone. The average lifespans were 78 weeks in treated males and 77 weeks in treated females, compared with 70 and 77 weeks in controls; 20/45 treated mice developed tumours (9 having lung adenomas), compared with 21/49 controls (13 having lung adenomas) (van Esch & Kroes, 1972).

Groups of 18 male and 18 female (C57BL/6xC3H/Anf)F$_1$ mice and 18 male and 18 female (C57BL/6xAKR)F$_1$ mice were given single s.c. injections of 1000 mg/kg bw commercial chloropropham (98.5% pure) in dimethyl sulphoxide on the 28th day of life and were observed until they were about 78 weeks of age, at which time 18, 18, 17 and 17 mice in the four groups, respectively, were still alive. Tumour incidences were compared with those in groups of 141, 154, 161 and 157 untreated or vehicle-injected controls that were necropsied. Incidences were not significantly increased (P>0.05) for any tumour type in any sex-strain subgroup or in the combined sexes of either strain (NTIS, 1968) [The Working Group noted that a negative result obtained with a single s.c. injection may not be an adequate basis for discounting carcinogenicity].

(c) Other experimental systems

In a two-stage skin carcinogenesis experiment, groups of 15 male and 15 female Swiss mice received chloropropham (m.p. 40-41°C; containing 30-40 mg/kg chloroaniline) either as a single dose of 15 mg in 1% tragacanth by stomach tube or the same dose weekly for 10 weeks or in the diet at a concentration of 1000 mg/kg of diet for 6 months. Promotion was induced by painting the skin with a 5% solution of croton oil in olive oil twice weekly for 6 months, starting either 3 days after the first administration of chloropropham by stomach tube or on the same day on which the diet containing chloropropham was given. Six months after the start of the experiment the numbers of mice with skin papillomas were: 1/22 in controls only painted with croton oil; 6/24 in mice given chloropropham by stomach tube once and croton oil; 2/26 in mice given chloropropham 10 times and croton oil; and 7/28 in mice fed chloropropham in the diet for 6 months and given croton oil. Tumour-bearing animals were observed for a further 10 months. A total of 40 papillomas appeared during the two periods (6 months of treatment + 10 months of observation); 7 of these were still present 6 months after the end of treatment. Two papillomas in the same

60

mouse had progressed to carcinomas by the end of the experiment. Only 1
tumour appeared in untreated controls. In the same experiment, 2 groups
of 15 male and 15 female Swiss mice were given 15 mg chloropropham in
tragacanth by stomach tube either once or 10 times over a period of 10 weeks.
A third group was fed 1000 mg chloropropham per kg of diet for 6 months.
All mice were killed 6 months after the beginning of the treatment. No skin
tumours appeared, and the incidence of lung adenomas was not increased
(van Esch et $al.$, 1958).

In a further experiment, a group of 50 female and 50 male Swiss mice
received 10 weekly administrations of 15 mg chloropropham in tragacanth by
stomach tube followed by twice weekly skin applications of croton oil for
26 weeks. There were no differences between treated and control animals
with regard to the number of papilloma-bearing animals, the total number
of papillomas or the proportion of regressing papillomas (van Esch et $al.$,
1965, reported in van Esch & Kroes, 1972).

3.2 Other relevant biological data

(a) Experimental systems

The acute oral LD_{50} of chloropropham was 10.39 g/kg bw in albino rats
fed diets containing 26% protein (as casein) and 1.20 g/kg bw in those
fed diets containing no protein (Boyd & Carsky, 1969).

After oral or i.p. administration of [^{14}C-isopropyl] and [^{14}C-ring-
labelled] chloropropham to rats, the 4-day urinary excretions were 50 and
85% of the dose, respectively, for the two sites of labelling; in the
case of the isopropyl-labelled compound, an additional 17-20% of the dose
was excreted as CO_2 via the lungs (Bobik et $al.$, 1972). There was no
significant difference in the rate or route of excretion among rats
receiving oral doses ranging from 4-200 mg/kg bw; the radioactivity was
distributed throughout the body, with highest concentrations in the kidneys
(Fang et $al.$, 1974). Hydrolysis of the carbamate linkage occurred in
neomycin-treated rats, and in $vitro$ investigations suggested that the
liver is the site of hydrolysis; 40% of an i.v. dose of chloropropham was
excreted in the 6-hour bile (Bobik et $al.$, 1972). When pregnant rats
were given ^{14}C-chloropropham, the radioactivity was readily transferred

to the foetuses, and its level did not decline in foetal tissues as rapidly as it did in the maternal organs. The pups of lactating rats that were given labelled chloropropham also contained radioactivity (Fang *et al.*, 1974).

In rats, the most important metabolic transformation of chloropropham (1) (Scheme 1) is hydroxylation in the *para*-position and conjugation of the resulting 4-hydroxychloropropham (2) with sulphate. Hydroxylation of the isopropyl residue accounts for about one-third of the metabolism of this herbicide. Approximately four times more monohydroxy compounds, (3) and (6), than dihydroxy compounds (8) were detected. Compound (6) undergoes further oxidation to yield the corresponding 1-carboxyethyl derivative (7). Hydrolytic fission of chloropropham yields *meta*-chloroaniline, carbon dioxide and isopropanol, which is further oxidized to acetone and carbon dioxide. Hydroxylation of the liberated *meta*-chloroaniline also takes place, to give *N*-acetyl-4-amino-2-chlorophenol (4) plus *N*-acetyl-2-amino-4-chlorophenol (5) (Aleksandrova & Klisenko, 1971a,b; Böhme & Grunow, 1969; Fang *et al.*, 1974; Grunow *et al.*, 1970; Kosyan, 1972).

Chloropropham inhibits spindle fibre formation and induces chromosome aberrations in plants (Nasta & Günther, 1973a; Stroev, 1970) and chlorophyll mutations in barley (Nasta & Günther, 1973b). Petite mutations were induced in *Saccharomyces cerevisiae* (Schubert, 1969); but no reverse mutations were detected in *Bacillus subtilis* (De Giovanni-Donnelly *et al.*, 1968) or in *Salmonella typhimurium* (Andersen *et al.*, 1972). Metabolic activation systems were not used in the tests in yeasts and bacteria.

(b) Man

No data were available to the Working Group.

3.3 Case reports and epidemiological studies

No data were available to the Working Group.

SCHEME 1

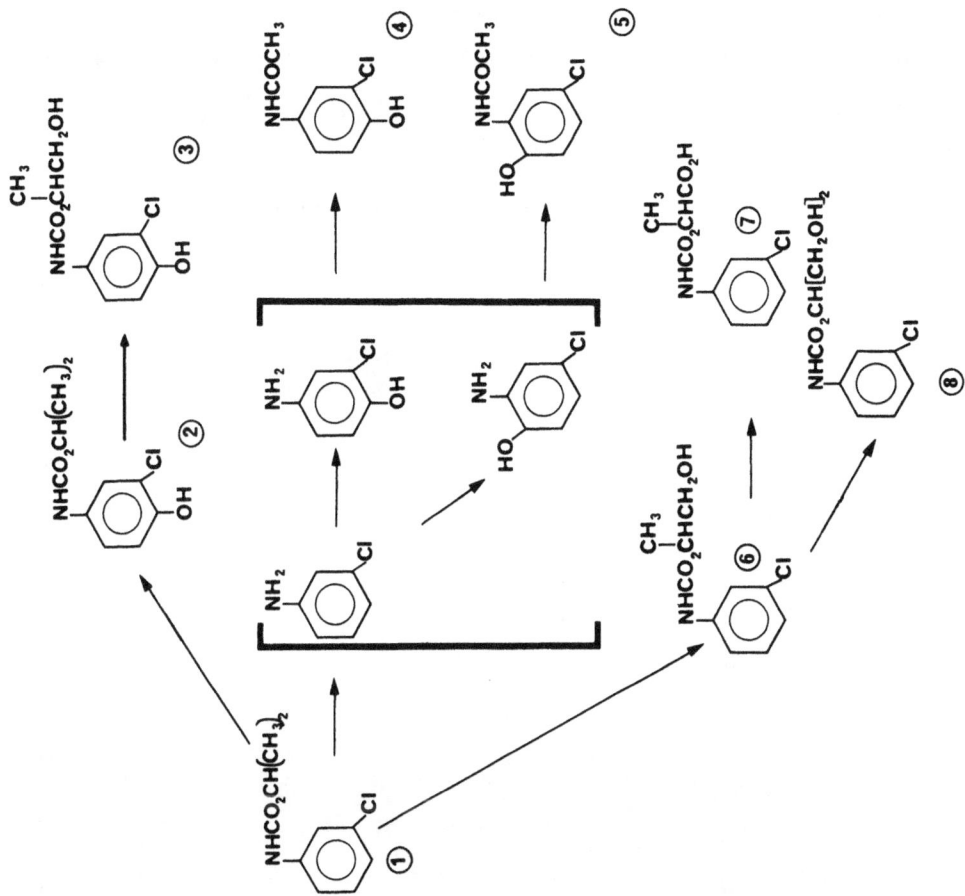

4. Comments on Data Reported and Evaluation

4.1 Animal data

Chloropropham produced no carcinogenic effects when administered orally to mice, rats and hamsters or subcutaneously to mice. Doses used in the studies in mice and hamsters did not necessarily correspond to the maximum tolerated doses.

In one experiment with oral administration in mice, chloropropham acted as an initiator of skin carcinogenesis. This was not confirmed in a subsequent experiment.

4.2 Human data

No case reports or epidemiological studies were available to the Working Group.

5. References

Aleksandrova, L.G. & Klisenko, M.A. (1971a) Metabolism of *N*-phenylcarbamic acid derivatives in warm-blooded animals. Gig. i Sanit., 36, 108-109

Aleksandrova, L.G. & Klisenko, M.A. (1971b) Identification of metabolic products of some derivatives of *N*-phenylcarbamic acid in warm-blooded animals. In: Tamm, O.M., ed., Proceedings of the 2nd All-Union Conference on the Studies on Residues of Pesticides and Prevention of their Pollution on Human and Animal Food and the Environment, Tallinn, 1970, Tallinn, Research Institute Epidemiological and Microbiological Hygiene, pp. 127-130

Andersen, K.J., Leighty, E.G. & Takahashi, M.T. (1972) Evaluation of herbicides for possible mutagenic properties. J. agric. Fd Chem., 20, 649-656

Berg, G.L., ed. (1975) Farm Chemicals Handbook 1975, Willoughby, Ohio, Meister

Bobik, A., Holder, G.M. & Ryan, A.J. (1972) Excretory and metabolic studies of isopropyl *N*-(3-chlorophenyl)carbamate in the rat. Fd Cosmet. Toxicol., 10, 163-170

Böhme, C. & Grunow, W. (1969) Über den Stoffwechsel von Carbamat-Herbiciden in der Ratte. I. Stoffwechsel des *m*-Chloranilins als Bestandteil von Chlorpropham und Barban. Fd Cosmet. Toxicol., 7, 125-133

Boyd, E.M. & Carsky, E. (1969) The acute oral toxicity of the herbicide chlorpropham in albino rats. Arch. environm. Hlth, 19, 621-627

Burge, W.D. & Gross, L.E. (1972) Determination of IPC, CIPC and propanil, and some metabolites of these herbicides in soil incubation studies. Soil Sci., 114, 440-443

California Department of Food and Agriculture (1975) Pesticide Use Report, 1974, Sacramento, p. 32

De Giovanni-Donnelly, R., Kolbye, S.M. & Greeves, P.D. (1968) The effects of IPC, CIPC, sevin and zectran on *Bacillus subtilis*. Experientia, 24, 80-81

Ercegovich, C.D. & Witkonton, S. (1972) An improved method for the analysis of residues of isopropyl *N*-(3-chlorophenyl)carbamate (chlorpropham) in alfalfa. J. agric. Fd Chem., 20, 344-347

van Esch, G.J. & Kroes, R. (1972) Long-term toxicity studies of chlorpropham and propham in mice and hamsters. Fd Cosmet. Toxicol., 10, 373-381

van Esch, G.J., van Genderen, H. & Vink, H.H. (1958) The production of skin tumours in mice by oral treatment with urethane, isopropyl-*N*-phenylcarbamate or isopropyl-*N*-chlorophenylcarbamate in combination with skin painting with croton oil and Tween 60. Brit. J. Cancer, 12, 355–362

Fang, S.C., Fallin, E., Montgomery, M.L. & Freed, V.H. (1974) Metabolic studies of ^{14}C-labeled propham and chlorpropham in the female rat. Pest. Biochem. Physiol., 4, 1–11

Fishbein, L. (1975) Chromatography of Environmental Hazards, Vol. 3, Pesticides, Amsterdam, Elsevier, pp. 624–626, 688–689

Fishbein, L. & Zielinski, W.L., Jr (1967) Chromatography of carbamates. Chromat. Rev., 9, 37–101

Frei, R.W. & Lawrence, J.F. (1973) Fluorigenic labelling in high-speed liquid chromatography. J. Chromat., 83, 321–330

Friestad, H.O. (1974) Rapid screening method, including automated colorimetry, for low residue levels of linuron and/or chlorpropham in vegetables. J. Ass. off. analyt. Chem., 57, 221–225

Gard, L.N. & Ferguson, C.E., Jr (1964) CIPC. In: Zweig, G., ed., Analytical Methods for Pesticides, Plant Growth Regulators and Food Additives, Vol. 4, Herbicides, New York, Academic Press, pp. 49–65

Grunow, W., Böhme, C. & Budczies, B. (1970) Über den Stoffwechsel von Carbamat-Herbiciden in der Ratte. II. Stoffwechsel von Chlorpropham und Barban. Fd Cosmet. Toxicol., 8, 277–288

Gutenmann, W.H. & Lisk, D.J. (1964) Electron affinity residue determination of CIPC, monuron, diuron, and linuron by direct hydrolysis and bromination. J. agric. Fd Chem., 12, 46–48

Innes, J.R.M., Ulland, B.M., Valerio, M.G., Petrucelli, L., Fishbein, L., Hart, E.R., Pallotta, A.J., Bates, R.R., Falk, H.L., Gart, J.J., Klein, M., Mitchell, I. & Peters, J. (1969) Bioassay of pesticides and industrial chemicals for tumorigenicity in mice: a preliminary note. J. nat. Cancer Inst., 42, 1101–1114

Japanese Ministry of Agriculture and Forestry (1975) Noyaku Yoran (Agricultural Chemicals Annual), 1975, Division of Plant Disease Prevention, Tokyo, Takeo Endo, pp. 38, 88, 95, 313

Kosyan, S.A. (1972) Metabolites of some phenylcarbamates in animals. In: Proceedings of the Conference on Toxicology and Hygiene of Mineral Oil Distillation Products, Yaroslavl, 1971, Vol. 2, Yaroslavl Medical Institute, pp. 110–115

Larson, P.S., Crawford, E.M., Blackwell Smith, R., Jr, Hennigar, G.R., Haag, H.B. & Finnegan, J.K. (1960) Chronic toxicologic studies on isopropyl *N*-(3-chlorophenyl)carbamate (CIPC). Toxicol. appl. Pharmacol., 2, 659-673

Lawrence, J.F. & Laver, G.W. (1974) Analysis of carbamate and urea herbicides in foods, using fluorogenic labeling. J. Ass. off. analyt. Chem., 57, 1022-1025

Lawrence, J.F. & Laver, G.W. (1975) Analysis of some carbamate and urea herbicides in foods by gas-liquid chromatography after alkylation. J. agric. Fd Chem., 23, 1106-1109

Nasta, A. & Günther, E. (1973a) Mitoseanomalien bei *Allium cepa* und *Hordeum vulgare* nach Einwirkung eines Carbamatherbizids. Biol. Zbl., 92, 27-36

Nasta, A. & Günther, E. (1973b) Häufigkeit von chlorophylldefekten Pflanzen nach Behandlung mit einem Carbamatherbizid und damit kombinierten Mutagenen bei *Hordeum vulgare*. Biol. Zbl., 92, 173-178

NTIS (National Technical Information Service) (1968) Evaluation of Carcinogenic, Teratogenic and Mutagenic Activities of Selected Pesticides and Industrial Chemicals, Vol. 1, Carcinogenic Study, Washington DC, US Department of Commerce

Schubert, A. (1969) Untersuchungen über die Induktion atmungsdefekter Hefemutanten durch chemische Pflanzenschutzmittel. II. Z. allg. Mikrobiol., 9, 483-485

Sherma, J. (1973) Chromatographic analysis of pesticide residues. CRC Crit. Rev. analyt. Chem., 3, 299-354

Stecher, P.G., ed. (1968) The Merck Index, 8th ed., Rahway, NJ, Merck & Co., p. 261

Still, G.G. & Mansager, E.R. (1973) Metabolism of isopropyl-3-chlorocarbanilate by cucumber plants. J. agric. Fd Chem., 21, 787-791

Stroev, V.S. (1970) The cytogenetic activity of the herbicides atrazine, chloro-IPC and paraquat. Genetika, 6, 31-37

Suzuki, K., Nagayoshi, H. & Kashiwa, T. (1974) The systematic separation and identification of pesticides in the second and third division. Agric. Biol. Chem., 38, 1433-1442

US Environmental Protection Agency (1974) EPA Compendium of Registered Pesticides, Washington DC, US Government Printing Office, pp. I-1-6.1-I-1-6.5

US Tariff Commission (1952) Synthetic Organic Chemicals, US Production and Sales, 1951, Second Series, Report No. 175, Washington DC, US Government Printing Office, p. 135

Weed Science Society of America (1974) *Herbicide Handbook*, 3rd ed.,
    Champaign, Illinois, pp. 101-106

Zweig, G. & Sherma, J. (1972) CIPC. In: Zweig, G., ed., *Analytical
    Methods for Pesticides and Plant Growth Regulators*, Vol. 6,
    Gas Chromatographic Analysis, New York, Academic Press, pp. 612-615

68

DIALLATE

1. Chemical and Physical Data

1.1 Synonyms and trade names

Chem. Abstr. Reg. Serial No.: 2303-16-4

Chem. Abstr. Name: Bis(1-methylethyl) carbamothioic acid, S-(2,3-dichloro-2-propenyl)ester

DATC; 2,3-DCDT; dichloroallyl diisopropylthiocarbamate; S-(2,3-dichloroallyl) diisopropylthiocarbamate; 2,3-dichloroallyl N,N-diisopropylthiolcarbamate; S-(2,3-dichloroallyl)-N,N-diisopropyl-thiolcarbamate; S-(2,3-dichloroallyl)diisopropylthiolcarbamate; 2,3-dichloro-2-propene-1-thiol, diisopropylcarbamate; diisopropyl-thiocarbamic acid, S-(2,3-dichloroallyl) ester

Avadex; CP 15336

1.2 Chemical formula and molecular weight

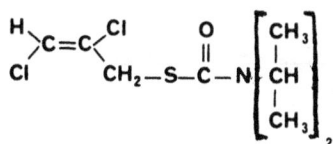   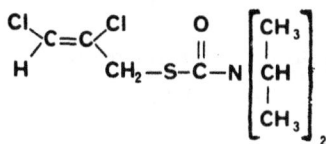

$trans$ isomer cis isomer

$C_{10}H_{17}Cl_2NOS$ Mol. wt: 270.2

1.3 Chemical and physical properties of the substance

From Stecher (1968) or Weed Science Society of America (1974), unless otherwise specified

(a) Description: Brown liquid

(b) Boiling-point: 150°C at 9 mm

(c) Melting-point: 25-30°C

(d) Density: $d^{25}_{15.6}$ 1.188

(e) Solubility: Slightly soluble in water (40 mg/l) at room temperature; soluble in acetone, benzene, chloroform, ether and heptane

(f) Volatility: Vapour pressure is 1.5×10^{-4} mm at 25°C. Evaporation rate is 10.63×10^{-9} mol/cm^2·hr at 20°C (Gueckel *et al.*, 1973).

1.4 Technical products and impurities

Diallate is available in the US as an emulsifiable concentrate containing 45% of the active ingredient and as a granular formulation containing 10% of the chemical (Weed Science Society of America, 1974). Commercial formulations of diallate contain roughly equal amounts of the *cis* and *trans* isomers (Rummens, 1975).

2. Production, Use, Occurrence and Analysis

For important background information on this section, see preamble, p. 15.

2.1 Production and use

Diallate can be prepared by reacting diisopropylamine with carbonyl sulphide and dichloropropene (Stecher, 1968).

It has been produced commercially in the US since 1961 (US Tariff Commission, 1962). The one company which produces it has recently announced considerable expansion of its capacity: a new manufacturing unit is being installed in the US, and an existing plant in Belgium is to be enlarged (Anon., 1975). Annual production of diallate in Europe is estimated to be in the range of 1 to 5 million kg.

The only known use for diallate is in the selective control of wild oats and other weeds in sugar beets, flax, barley, corn, forage legumes, lentils, peas, potatoes, soyabeans, root crops, oil crops, fruit trees and ornamentals (Weed Science Society of America, 1974). Diallate is registered in the US for pre-planting or pre-emergence incorporation in soil for 11 agricultural crops, largely forage or field crops. Less than 100 thousand kg

70

were used on all agricultural crops in the US in 1971.

A residue tolerance of 0.05 mg/kg has been established in the US for
these crops (US Environmental Protection Agency, 1972). The residue
tolerance in Europe is of the order of 0.1 mg/kg.

2.2 Occurrence

Diallate is not known to occur as a natural product. It has an average
half-life of about 30 days in soil when applied at recommended rates (1.5-
3.5 pounds/acre) (Weed Science Society of America, 1974). Residual amounts
may occur on or in treated crops after harvesting.

2.3 Analysis

A thin-layer chromatography method for systematic separation and
detection of sixty-one pesticides, including diallate, has been described;
the limit of detection for diallate was 0.5 µg or 2.0 µg, depending on
the system employed (Ebing, 1972). Preparative gas-liquid chromatography
was used in one study to separate the *cis* and *trans* isomers of diallate
for identification by techniques such as nuclear magnetic resonance
and infra-red spectrometry (Rummens, 1975).

3. Biological Data Relevant to the Evaluation
of Carcinogenic Risk to Man

3.1 Carcinogenicity and related studies in animals

(a) Oral administration

Mouse: Groups of 18 male and 18 female (C57BL/6xC3H/Anf)F_1 mice and
18 male and 18 female (C57BL/6xAKR)F_1 mice received commercial diallate
(b.p. 145-150°C at 9 mm) according to the following schedule: 215 mg/kg bw
in gelatine at 7 days of age by stomach tube and the same amount (not
adjusted for increasing body weight) daily up to 4 weeks of age; subsequently,
the mice were given 560 mg diallate per kg of diet. The dose was the maximum
tolerated dose for infant and young mice but not necessarily so for adults.
The experiment was terminated when the animals were about 78 weeks of age,
at which time 15, 16, 16 and 14 mice in the four groups, respectively, were
still alive. Tumour incidences were compared with those observed among

79-90 necropsied mice of each sex and strain, which either had been untreated or had received gelatine only. The incidence of hepatomas in necropsied male (C57BL/6xC3H/Anf)F$_1$ mice was 13/16, compared with 8/79 in controls; that in necropsied male (C57BL/6xAKR)F$_1$ mice was 10/18, compared with 5/90 in controls [P<0.001]. The incidences of hepatomas among females were 3/16 in the first strain, compared with 0/87 in controls, and 1/15 in the second, compared with 1/82 in controls [P>0.05]. In addition, 4/16 (C57BL/6xC3H/Anf)F$_1$ male mice died with lung adenomas, compared with 5/79 controls [P>0.05] (Innes *et al.*, 1969; NTIS, 1968).

Rat: Results of a 2-year feeding study with diallate in Charles River CD rats were reported briefly (Ulland *et al.*, 1973) [The inadequate reporting does not allow an evaluation of this experiment].

(b)   Subcutaneous administration

Mouse: Groups of 18 male and 18 female (C57BL/6xC3H/Anf)F$_1$ mice and 18 male and 18 female (C57BL/6xAKR)F$_1$ mice were given single s.c. injections of 1000 mg/kg bw commercial diallate (b.p. 146-150°C at 9 mm) in corn oil on the 28th day of life and were observed until they were about 78 weeks of age, at which time 17, 18, 18 and 15 mice in the four groups, respectively, were still alive. Tumour incidences were compared with those in groups of 141, 154, 161 and 157 untreated or vehicle-injected controls that were necropsied. Systemic reticulum-cell sarcomas developed in 4/18 necropsied male (C57BL/6xC3H/Anf)F$_1$ mice, compared with 8/141 control males of that strain (P<0.05). Such tumours were not observed in treated males of the second strain (NTIS, 1968).

3.2   Other relevant biological data

(a)   Experimental systems

Oral LD$_{50}$ values for diallate in rats range from 393-1000 mg/kg bw; the dermal LD$_{50}$ in rabbits is 2000-2500 mg/kg bw (Ben-Dyke *et al.*, 1970). In mice, rats and cats, injection of diallate caused central nervous system excitation, which progressed within a few minutes to depression and clonic-tonic convulsions (Pestova, 1966).

72

Repeated application of diallate to the eyes and skin of guinea-pigs and rabbits caused local irritation, which was followed by loss of weight, neutrophile leucocytosis, eosinopenia and erythropenia; oral and subcutaneous administration produced similar effects (Doloshitsky, 1969; Gzhegotsky & Doloshitsky, 1971).

Tests for reverse mutations in *Salmonella typhimurium* strains were negative for base substitution and frame-shift mutations (Andersen *et al.*, 1972); metabolic activation systems were not used in these tests.

(b) Man

No data were available to the Working Group.

3.3 Case reports and epidemiological studies

No data were available to the Working Group.

4. Comments on Data Reported and Evaluation[1]

4.1 Animal data

Diallate is carcinogenic in mice after its oral administration: it produced an increased incidence of liver-cell tumours in males of two strains and a slight increase in the number of liver-cell tumours in females of one strain. A single subcutaneous injection in mice produced a slight increase in the incidence of systemic reticulum-cell sarcomas in males of one strain.

4.2 Human data

No case reports or epidemiological studies were available to the Working Group.

---

[1]See also the section, 'Animal data in relation to the evaluation of risk to man' in the introduction to this volume, p. 13.

5. References

Andersen, K.J., Leighty, E.G. & Takahashi, M.T. (1972) Evaluation of herbicides for possible mutagenic properties. J. agric. Fd Chem., 20, 649-656

Anon. (1975) It's news to me. Fertilizer Solutions, January-February, p. 107

Ben-Dyke, R., Sanderson, D.M. & Noakes, D.N. (1970) Acute toxicity data for pesticides. Wld Rev. Pest. Contr., 9, 119-127

Doloshitsky, S.L. (1969) Hygienic standardization of herbicide avadex containing chlorine in water. Gig. i Sanit., 34, 21-28

Ebing, W. (1972) Routinemethode zur dünnschichtchromatographischen Identifizierung der Pestizidrückstände aus der Klassen der Triazine, Carbamate, Harnstoffe und Uracile. J. Chromat., 65, 533-545

Glueckel, W., Synnatschke, G. & Rittig, R. (1973) A method for determining the volatility of active ingredients used in plant protection. Pest. Sci., 4, 137-147

Gzhegotsky, M.I. & Doloshitsky, S.L. (1971) Skin resorption effect of herbicides. Vrach. Delo, 11, 133-134

Innes, J.R.M., Ulland, B.M., Valerio, M.G., Petrucelli, L., Fishbein, L., Hart, E.R., Pallotta, A.J., Bates, R.R., Falk, H.L., Gart, J.J., Klein, M., Mitchell, I. & Peters, J. (1969) Bioassay of pesticides and industrial chemicals for tumorigenicity in mice: a preliminary note. J. nat. Cancer Inst., 42, 1101-1114

NTIS (National Technical Information Service) (1968) Evaluation of Carcinogenic, Teratogenic and Mutagenic Activities of Selected Pesticides and Industrial Chemicals, Vol. 1, Carcinogenic Study, Washington DC, US Department of Commerce

Pestova, A.G. (1966) Toxicity of diptal and avadex. Gig. Toksikol. Pest. Klin. Oltravleny, 4, 166-169

Rummens, F.H.A. (1975) Separation and structural assignment of the cis and trans isomers of S-(2,3-dichloroallyl)diisopropylthiocarbamate (diallate). Weed Sci., 23, 7-10

Stecher, P.G., ed. (1968) The Merck Index, 8th ed., Rahway, NJ, Merck & Co., p. 337

Ulland, B., Weisburger, E.K. & Weisburger, J.H. (1973) Chronic toxicity and carcinogenicity of industrial chemicals and pesticides. Toxicol. appl. Pharmacol., 25, 446

US Environmental Protection Agency (1972) EPA Compendium of Registered Pesticides, Washington DC, US Government Printing Office, pp. I-D-18.1 - I-D-18.2

US Tariff Commission (1962) Synthetic Organic Chemicals, US Production and Sales, 1961, TC Publication 72, Washington DC, US Government Printing Office, p. 167

Weed Science Society of America (1974) Herbicide Handbook, 3rd ed., Champaign, Illinois, p. 136

DIMETHYLCARBAMOYL CHLORIDE

1. Chemical and Physical Data

1.1 Synonyms and trade names

Chem. Abstr. Reg. Serial No.: 79-44-7

Chem. Abstr. Name: Dimethylcarbamic chloride

(Dimethylamino)carbonyl chloride; dimethylcarbamic acid chloride; dimethylcarbamidoyl chloride; dimethyl carbamoyl chloride; N,N-dimethylcarbamoyl chloride; dimethylcarbamyl chloride; N,N-dimethyl-carbamyl chloride

1.2 Chemical formula and molecular weight

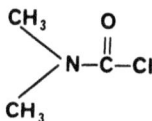

$$\begin{array}{c} CH_3 \quad\quad O \\ \diagdown \quad \| \\ N-C-Cl \\ \diagup \\ CH_3 \end{array}$$

C_3H_6ClNO Mol. wt: 107.6

1.3 Chemical and physical properties of the substance

(a) Description: Liquid

(b) Boiling-point: 47-49°C at 12 mm (Hasserodt, 1968); 64°C at 20 mm (Birkofer & Krebs, 1968)

(c) Melting-point: -33°C (von Hey $et\ al.$, 1974)

(d) Density: d_4^{20} 1.1678 (Prager & Jacobson, 1922)

(e) Refractive index: n_D^{20} 1.4529 (Hasserodt, 1968)

(f) Stability: Rapidly hydrolyses in water to dimethylamine, carbon dioxide and hydrogen chloride; its half-life at 0°C is about 6 minutes (Van Duuren $et\ al.$, 1972)

1.4 Technical products and impurities

No data were available to the Working Group.

2. Production, Use, Occurrence and Analysis

For important background information on this section, see preamble, p. 15.

2.1 Production and use

Michler & Escherich (1879) first reported preparation of dimethyl-carbamoyl chloride by the reaction of dimethylamine with phosgene, and this process is believed to be used currently for its commercial production.

Dimethylcarbamoyl chloride was produced in the US between 1958 (US Tariff Commission, 1959) and 1971 (US Tariff Commission, 1973). Although there were five US manufacturers producing this chemical in the past, there is now only one, who makes less than 450 kg per year.

The manufacture of dimethylcarbamoyl chloride was begun in the Federal Republic of Germany in 1961, and approximately 120 thousand kg are produced each year (von Hey *et al.*, 1974). It is also manufactured and used in the UK (Anon., 1975a).

The only known use of dimethylcarbamoyl chloride is as a chemical intermediate in the production of drugs and pesticides. Dimethylcarbamoyl chloride-derived parasympathomimetic (cholinergic) agents being used for treatment of myasthenia gravis in the US are: pyridostigmine bromide (mestinon bromide; 3-hydroxy-1-methylpyridinium bromide dimethylcarbamate); neostigmine bromide (3-dimethylcarbamoxyphenyl trimethylammonium bromide); and neostigmine methylsulphate (3-dimethylcarbamoxyphenyl trimethylammonium methyl sulphate).

The dimethylcarbamoyl chloride-derived pesticides approved by the US Environmental Protection Agency for use in the US are: the herbicide, tandex [*meta*-(3,3-dimethylureido)phenyl-*tert*-butylcarbamate] (Johnson, 1972); the insecticide, dimetilan (2-dimethylcarbamoyl-3-methyl-5-pyrazolyl dimethylcarbamate) (US Environmental Protection Agency, 1972); and the aphicide, pirimor (pirimicarb; 5,6-dimethyl-2-dimethylamino-4-pyrimidinyl dimethyl carbamate) (Anon., 1975b).

Several dimethylcarbamoyl chloride-derived pesticides are not approved by the US Environmental Protection Agency for use in the US but are believed to be used elsewhere; these are: isolan (1-isopropyl-3-methyl-5-pyrazolyl dimethylcarbamate); pyrolan (1-phenyl-3-methyl-5-pyrazolyldimethylcarbamate); and dimetan (5,5-dimethyldihydroresorcinol dimethylcarbamate).

2.2 Occurrence

Dimethylcarbamoyl chloride is not known to occur as a natural product.

In one manufacturing plant in the Federal Republic of Germany, the production of dimethylcarbamoyl chloride is carried out in a closed system; during evacuation and cleaning, workers wear respirators and gloves. Concentrations of up to 1.5 ppm (7 mg/m^3) have been reported in the air (von Hey *et al.*, 1974). It is possible that levels of exposure might be considerably higher in facilities in which the chemical is used for further synthesis. In any such situation where closed systems are not used a potential exposure may exist for both workers and the community.

2.3 Analysis

In one method dimethylcarbamoyl chloride was reacted with 4-(*para*-nitrobenzyl)pyridine in a triethylamine-methylethyl ketone solvent for 8 hours at 50°C. The resulting product was analysed spectrophotometrically (Agree & Meeker, 1966). A more sensitive method to detect levels as low as 17 ppb in the air, using acetone as the solvent, has been reported (Rusch *et al.*, 1976).

Gas chromatography has been used to measure atmospheric levels in working environments. Levels as low as 0.06 ppm (0.3 mg/m^3) were reported, but no indication was given as to the lower limit of sensitivity of the method (von Hey *et al.*, 1974).

3. Biological Data Relevant to the Evaluation of Carcinogenic Risk to Man

3.1 Carcinogenicity and related studies in animals

(a) Skin application

Mouse: Of 50 female ICR/Ha Swiss mice given 2 mg dimethylcarbamoyl chloride (b.p. 84°C at 50 mm) in 0.1 ml acetone on the interscapular region thrice weekly during 492 days, 40 developed skin papillomas (persisting at

79

least 30 days); of these, 30 progressed to skin carcinomas. The median survival time was 386 days, compared with 543 days in 50 controls receiving acetone only. No tumours at other sites are mentioned in this paper (Van Duuren *et al.*, 1974); however, in a preliminary report of the same study, 2/26 treated and 0/9 control animals dying before 385 days had papillary tumours of the lungs (Van Duuren *et al.*, 1972).

Of 30 female ICR/Ha Swiss mice given a single application of 2 mg dimethylcarbamoyl chloride in 0.1 ml acetone followed 2 weeks later by 3 applications per week of 2.5 µg phorbol myristyl acetate (PMA) in 0.1 ml acetone for the duration of the experiment (more than 385 days), 6 developed skin papillomas, the first appearing 79 days after the start of PMA treatment. Papillomas occurred in 3/30 controls receiving PMA only, the first tumour appearing at 224 days, and in 0/30 mice given a single application of dimethylcarbamoyl chloride (Van Duuren *et al.*, 1974).

(b) Subcutaneous administration

Mouse: Of 50 female ICR/Ha Swiss mice given weekly s.c. injections of 5 mg dimethylcarbamoyl chloride (b.p. 84°C at 50 mm) in 0.05 ml tricaprylin for 26 weeks, 36 developed local sarcomas, and 3 had local squamous-cell carcinomas. The median survival time was 280 days, compared with 493 days in controls receiving solvent alone. Of 50 controls, 1 developed a sarcoma (P<0.01), and none had carcinomas. No tumours at other sites are mentioned in this report, even though animals were autopsied completely except for the cranial region (Van Duuren *et al.*, 1974); however, in a preliminary report of the same study, of 47/50 treated and 4/30 control animals dying before 385 days, 4 of the treated group and 0 of the control group had papillary tumours of the lungs (Van Duuren *et al.*, 1972).

(c) Intraperitoneal administration

Mouse: Of 30 female ICR/Ha Swiss mice given weekly i.p. injections of 1 mg dimethylcarbamoyl chloride in 0.05 ml tricaprylin for up to 450 days (end of the experiment), 14 developed papillary tumours of the lungs, compared with 10/30 mice given tricaprylin alone and with 29/100 untreated mice. Eight treated mice and 1 control given the solvent alone developed local sarcomas, and 1 treated mouse developed a squamous-cell carcinoma of the skin (Van Duuren *et al.*, 1974).

3.2 Other relevant biological data

(a) Experimental systems

In mice, the i.p. LD_{50} is approximately 350 mg/kg bw; in rats, the oral LD_{50} for dimethylcarbamoyl chloride in oil is approximately 1170 mg/kg bw (von Hey *et al.*, 1974).

Rats tolerated an 8-minute exposure to an atmosphere saturated at $20^{\circ}C$ with dimethylcarbamoyl chloride and survived 14 days post-exposure; but when animals were exposed for 1 or 2 hours, 5/6 or 6/6 died, respectively. Dimethylcarbamoyl chloride damages mucous membranes of the nose, throat and lungs and causes difficulty in breathing, sometimes only after several days. Skin application of undiluted dimethylcarbamoyl chloride to rats and rabbits produced skin irritation, with subsequent degeneration of the epidermis and outer dermal structures; skin-sensitization tests in guinea-pigs were negative. Conjunctivitis and keratitis occurred in irritation tests in rabbit's eyes (von Hey *et al.*, 1974).

Dimethylcarbamoyl chloride behaves as a direct-acting acylating carcinogen, which is consistent with the production *in vivo* of the corresponding carbonium ion (Van Duuren *et al.*, 1972).

Dimethylcarbamoyl chloride (5.3 mg) induced reverse mutations in *Salmonella typhimurium* strains TA1535 and TA100; no metabolic activation was required (McCann *et al.*, 1975).

(b) Man

One case of eye irritation and one of liver disturbances have been observed in workers exposed to dimethylcarbamoyl chloride (von Hey *et al.*, 1974).

3.3 Case reports and epidemiological studies

No cancer deaths (out of a total of 6 deaths) or X-ray indications of lung cancer were reported in an investigation of 39 dimethylcarbamoyl chloride production workers (3 of whom were females), 26 processing workers and 42 ex-workers, aged 17-65 and exposed for periods ranging from 6 months to 12 years (von Hey *et al.*, 1974).

4. Comments on Data Reported and Evaluation[1]

4.1 Animal data

Dimethylcarbamoyl chloride is carcinogenic in mice by skin application or by subcutaneous or intraperitoneal injection: it produced local tumours by each of the three routes of administration.

4.2 Human data

The available epidemiological study is inadequate to assess the carcinogenicity of this compound in man.

---

[1]See also the section, 'Animal data in relation to the evaluation of risk to man' in the introduction to this volume, p. 13.

5. References

Agree, A.M. & Meeker, R.L. (1966) Quantitative determination of micro and semi-micro concentrations of acylating agents by 4-(p-nitrobenzyl) pyridine reagent. Talanta, 13, 1151-1160

Anon. (1975a) In brief. Chemical Age, January 24, p. 19

Anon. (1975b) 1975 Pesticide roundup. Farm Chemicals, 138, 50

Birkofer, L. & Krebs, K. (1968) N,N-Disubstituierte Carbamoyl- und Thiocarbamoylchloride über Silyl-Derivate. Tetrahedron Lett., 7, 885-888

Hasserodt, U. (1968) Die Reaktion von Schwefeldichlorid, Dischwefeldichlorid und Sulfurylchlorid mit (Thio)Amiden zu (Thio)Carbamidsäurechloriden und Senfölen. Chem. Ber., 101, 113-120

von Hey, W., Thiess, A.M. & Zeller, H. (1974) Zur Frage etwaiger Gesundheitsschädigungen bei der Herstellung und Verarbeitung von Dimethylcarbaminsäurechlorid. Zbl. Arbeitsmed., 24, 71-77

Johnson, O. (1972) Pesticides 1972. II. Chemical Week, July 26

McCann, J., Spingarn, N.E., Kobori, J. & Ames, B.N. (1975) Detection of carcinogens as mutagens: bacterial tester strains with R factor plasmids. Proc. nat. Acad. Sci. (Wash.), 72, 979-983

Michler, W. & Escherich, C. (1879) Concerning multiple-substituted ureas. Chem. Ber., 12, 1162-1164

Prager, B. & Jacobson, P., eds (1922) Beilsteins Handbuch der organischen Chemie, 4th ed., Vol. 4, Syst. No. 335, Berlin, Springer-Verlag, p. 73

Rusch, G.M., La Mendola, S.L., Katz, G.V. & Laskin, S. (1976) Determination of low levels of dimethylcarbamoyl chloride in air. Analyt. Chem. (in press)

US Environmental Protection Agency (1972) EPA Compendium of Registered Pesticides, Vol. III, Insecticides, Acaricides, Molluscicides, and Antifouling Compounds, Washington DC, US Government Printing Office, p. III-H-5

US Tariff Commission (1959) Synthetic Organic Chemicals, US Production and Sales, 1958, Report No. 205, Second Series, Washington DC, US Government Printing Office, p. 145

US Tariff Commission (1973) Synthetic Organic Chemicals, US Production and Sales, 1971, TC Publication 614, Washington DC, US Government Printing Office, p. 218

Van Duuren, B.L., Goldschmidt, B.M., Katz, C. & Seidman, I. (1972)
Dimethylcarbamyl chloride, a multipotential carcinogen. J. nat. Cancer
Inst., 48, 1539-1541

Van Duuren, B.L., Goldschmidt, B.M., Katz, C., Seidman, I. & Paul, J.S.
(1974) Carcinogenic activity of alkylating agents. J. nat. Cancer
Inst., 53, 695-700

DISULFIRAM*

1. Chemical and Physical Data

1.1 Synonyms and trade names

Chem. Abstr. Reg. Serial No.: 97-77-8

Chem. Abstr. Name: Tetraethylthioperoxydicarbonic diamide

Bis[(diethylamino)thioxomethyl] disulphide; bis(diethylthiocarbamoyl) disulphide; bis(N,N-diethylthiocarbamoyl) disulphide; disulphuram; 1,1'-dithiobis(N,N-diethylthioformamide); ethyl thiram; ethyl thiurad; TATD; TETD; tetraethylthiram disulphide; tetraethylthiuram; tetra-ethylthiuram disulphide; N,N,N',N'-tetraethylthiuram disulphide; tetraethylthiuran disulphide; TTD

Abstensil; Abstinyl; Alcophobin; Antabus; Antabuse; Antadix; Antethyl; Antalcol; Antietanol; Antietil; Antikol; Aversan; Contralin; Cronetal; Ekagom TEDS; Esperal; Etabus; Ethyl tuads; Ethyl Tuex; Exhorran; Noxal; Refusal; Stopetyl; Tetradine; Tetraetil; Thiuram E; Thiuranide

1.2 Chemical formula and molecular weight

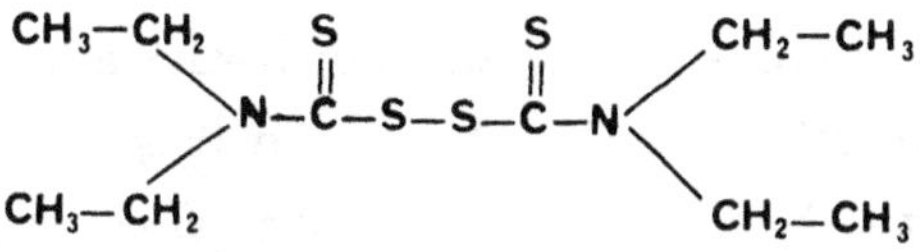

$C_{10}H_{20}N_2S_4$ Mol. wt: 296.5

1.3 Chemical and physical properties of the pure substance

(a) Description: Yellowish-white crystals (Stecher, 1968)

(b) Melting-point: 70°C (Stecher, 1968); 71-72°C (Weast, 1975)

---

*Much of the information on the carcinogenicity of this substance refers to the rubber-processing grade chemical.

(c) Spectroscopy data: For infra-red and nuclear magnetic resonance
spectral data, see Grasselli (1973).

(d) Solubility: At 25°C, soluble in water (0.02 g/100 ml), ethanol
(3.82 g/100 ml), ether (7.14 g/100 ml); also soluble in acetone,
benzene, chloroform and carbon disulphide (Stecher, 1968)

1.4 Technical products and impurities

Disulfiram is available in the US for rubber processing with the
following typical specifications: physical state, cubes; colour, buff to
light grey; density, 1.27 ± 0.03; melting range, 63-75°C; ash, 0.5% max.;
moisture, 1.0% max.; available sulphur, 10.8% (Anon., 1973, 1975). It is
also available in a dispersion containing 25-30% binder and in a 50:50
mixture with thiram (methyl tuads) (Anon., 1975). For medicinal purposes,
a pharmaceutical grade of disulfiram is available as tablets containing up
to 500 mg (Anon., 1976).

2. Production, Use, Occurrence and Analysis

For important background information on this section, see preamble,
p. 15.

2.1 Production and use

The first reported preparation of disulfiram was by the addition of
iodine to an ethanolic solution of the diethylamine salt of diethyldithiocarbamic acid (Grodzki, 1881). It can be prepared by adding sulphuric acid
and hydrogen peroxide to an aqueous solution of sodium diethyldithiocarbamate
(Shaver, 1968), or by treating sodium diethyldithiocarbamate with sodium
hypochlorite (Bailey, 1931).

Commercial production of disulfiram in the US was first reported in
1940 (US Tariff Commission, 1941), and three manufacturers reported
production in 1974 (US International Trade Commission, 1975). It is also
produced in the Benelux countries, France, Italy and the UK. World production of disulfiram is estimated to be from 510 to 550 thousand kg per year.

The major use of disulfiram is as an accelerator in compounding natural,
styrene-butadiene, isobutylene-isoprene and Neoprene W rubbers. It is

fast-curing, non-discolouring and non-staining and can be used with or without sulphur. It can be used as a primary or secondary accelerator with aldehyde amines and guanidines and is also used as a cure retarder in chloroprene and Neoprene G rubbers (Anon., 1975).

Pharmaceutical grade disulfiram is used in aversion therapy for chronic alcoholism (Anon., 1976). Threatment consists generally of a single dose of 0.5 g during 1-2 weeks, then 0.25 g/day. It is estimated that less than 5 thousand kg disulfiram are used in human medicine in the US annually.

Although disulfiram may have been used as a pesticide, it has not been approved for that use in the US by the Environmental Protection Agency.

In 1975, the American Conference of Government Industrial Hygienists set 2 mg/m^3 as a trial threshold limit value for disulfiram in the workplace air over any eight-hour workshift for a forty-hour work week (ACGIH, 1975).

2.2 Occurrence

Disulfiram is not known to occur as a natural product.

2.3 Analysis

Methods for the chromatographic analysis of carbamates, including disulfiram, have been reviewed (Fishbein & Zielinski, 1967).

When heated with sulphuric acid, disulfiram is quantitatively converted to carbon disulphide, which can be determined as copper diethyldithiocarbamate. Differential cathode ray polarography has been used to estimate disulfiram in human blood; 85 to 105% was recovered from 1 ml of citrated whole human blood containing 1.0 to 30 μg. The carbon disulphide present in the exhaled air of patients treated with disulfiram may be determined similarly (Brown *et al.*, 1974). A similar procedure was used to determine the presence of disulfiram added to urine; recoveries were 85-95% (Porter & Williams, 1972). A gas chromatographic method for the determination of carbon disulphide in the exhaled air of disulfiram-treated patients has been described (Wells & Koves, 1974).

87

3. Biological Data Relevant to the Evaluation of Carcinogenic Risk to Man

3.1 Carcinogenicity and related studies in animals

(a) Oral administration

Mouse: Groups of 18 male and 18 female (C57BL/6xC3H/Anf)F_1 mice and 18 male and 18 female (C57BL/6xAKR)F_1 mice received commercial disulfiram (rubber-processing grade; m.p. 63-75°C) according to the following schedule: 100 mg/kg bw in gelatine at 7 days of age by stomach tube and the same amount (not adjusted for increasing body weight) daily up to 4 weeks of age; subsequently, the mice were given 323 mg per kg of diet. The dose was the maximum tolerated dose for infant and young mice but not necessarily so for adults. The experiment was terminated when the animals were about 78 weeks of age, at which time 15, 18, 7 and 15 mice in the four groups, respectively, were still alive. Tumour incidences were compared with those observed among 79-90 necropsied mice of each strain and sex, which either had been untreated or had received gelatine only. An excess number of tumour-bearing animals was found among males of both strains (first strain, 10/17 necropsied *versus* 22/79 controls [P<0.02]; second strain, 13/16 necropsied *versus* 16/90 controls [P<0.001]). In males of the first strain, pulmonary adenomas were found in 5/17, compared with 5/79 in controls (P<0.01), and hepatomas in 8/17, compared with 8/79 in controls (P<0.001). In males of the second strain, only subcutaneous fibrosarcomas were found in excess and were present in 10/16 necropsied mice (Innes *et al*., 1969; NTIS, 1968). [The occurrence of a substantial number of subcutaneous sarcomas in mice following the oral administration of a chemical is extremely unusual in chemical carcinogenesis experiments. This observation raises some doubts as to the significance of the above finding].

Rat: A group of 40 14-week old Sprague-Dawley male rats was given an aqueous solution of commercial disulfiram by stomach tube twice weekly for an unspecified number of weeks; the weekly dose was 500 mg/kg bw. Mean survival time was 65 weeks. Two animals developed a benign interstitial-cell tumour of the testis; no other tumours were observed. Among 600 untreated control rats, whose mean survival time was 98 weeks, 38 developed a total of 42 tumours at different sites (Schmähl *et al.*, 1976) [The Working Group noted the inadequate duration of this experiment].

(b) Subcutaneous administration

Mouse: Groups of 18 male and 18 female $(C57BL/6xC3H/Anf)F_1$ mice and 18 male and 18 female $(C57BL/6xAKR)F_1$ mice were given single s.c. injections of 1000 mg/kg bw commercial disulfiram (rubber-processing grade; m.p. 63-75°C) in 0.5% gelatine at 28 days of age and were observed until they were about 78 weeks of age, at which time 15, 17, 18, and 18 mice in the four groups, respectively, were still alive. Tumour incidences were compared with those in groups of 141, 154, 161 and 157 untreated or vehicle-injected controls that were necropsied. An increased incidence of reticulum-cell sarcomas was found in 3/18 females of the second strain, compared with 5/157 controls [P<0.05] (NTIS, 1968).

3.2 Other relevant biological data

(a) Experimental systems

Only minimal signs of toxicity were seen in mice administered up to 10 g/kg bw disulfiram orally. Oral LD_{50}'s in rats, rabbits and dogs ranged from 2-10 g/kg bw. Major signs of severe toxicity were ataxia, hypothermia and flaccid paralysis (Child & Crump, 1952). In rats, concentrations of 100-2500 mg per kg of diet were given for up to 2 years; toxic effects occurred only at the highest concentration, at as early as 8 weeks (Fitzhugh *et al.*, 1952). Other investigations showed that chronic dosing with 1000-2000 mg/kg of diet with disulfiram retards the growth and reproductive capacity of rats and decreases longevity (Holck *et al.*, 1970). Doses of 25-500 mg/kg bw disulfiram have anti-thyroid properties (Christensen & Wase, 1954).

In rats, the following metabolites of disulfiram were found: diethyl-dithiocarbamate, diethyldithiocarbamate *S*-glucuronide, inorganic sulphate, diethylamine and carbon disulphide. A small amount of the S was bound to proteins as mixed disulphides. After i.p. injection of 10 mg, 8% of the -SH groups of plasma proteins and about 0.1-0.2% of the -SH groups of the soluble liver proteins were blocked (Strömme, 1963, 1965). Disulfiram has been shown to inhibit the activity of aldehyde dehydrogenase, resulting in acetaldehyde accumulation (Hald & Jacobsen, 1948), of dopamine β-hydroxylase (Goldstein, 1966), hexokinase (Strömme, 1963), glyceraldehyde 3-phosphate dehydrogenase (Nygaard & Sumner, 1952), xanthine oxidase (Richert et al., 1950) and D-amino acid oxidase (Neims et al., 1966) and to depress cytochrome P-450 levels (Zemaitis & Greene, 1976).

The mechanism of disulfiram-ethanol interaction in vivo is incompletely understood (van Logten, 1972). Thus, disulfiram (Hald et al., 1949; Larsen, 1948), or one of its metabolites, diethyldithiocarbamate (Domar et al., 1949; Eldjarn, 1950a) or carbon disulphide (Johnston & Prickett, 1952; Prickett & Johnson, 1953), may interfere with normal ethanol metabolism and so give rise to toxic amounts of intermediary products (Hald et al., 1949; Larsen, 1948). On the other hand, ethanol may interfere with the catabolism of disulfiram to make it more toxic (Strömme, 1963).

The acute toxicity of N-nitrosodimethylamine in rats and mice and the N-7-methylation of guanine in liver DNA were reduced by simultaneous administration of disulfiram (Schmähl et al., 1971).

The inhibitory effect of disulfiram on carcinogenesis has been demonstrated for benzo(a)pyrene-induced forestomach tumours in mice (Wattenberg, 1974), for 1,2-dimethylhydrazine-induced large-intestine tumours in mice (Wattenberg, 1975), for dimethylbenzanthracene-induced mammary tumours in rats (Wattenberg, 1974) and for N-nitrosodimethyl- and N-nitrosodiethylamine-induced liver tumours in rats but not for other tumours induced by these nitrosamines (Schmähl et al., 1976).

Disulfiram can react with nitrite to form N-nitrosodiethylamine (Lijinsky et al., 1972).

(b) Man

The metabolism of disulfiram in man is similar to that in animals (Asmussen et al., 1948a,b; Eldjarn, 1950b; Hald & Jacobsen, 1948; Hald et al., 1948; Kaslander, 1963; Merlevede & Casier, 1961). Strömme's observation (Strömme, 1965) that ethanol interferes with the catabolism of disulfiram also applies in man.

Lilly (1975) has examined chromosomes from alcoholics treated with total doses of disulfiram ranging from 0.6-93 g per person. No increase in the number of chromosome aberrations was found. Tests *in vitro* on cultured lymphocytes with 10^{-4}-10^{-8} M disulfiram also revealed no effect on the chromosomes.

3.3 Case reports and epidemiological studies

No data were available to the Working Group.

4. Comments on Data Reported and Evaluation

4.1 Animal data

Disulfiram (of rubber-processing grade) was tested by oral administration and by single subcutaneous injection in two strains of mice. When given by the oral route it increased the incidence of liver-cell tumours and caused a slight increase in the number of lung tumours in males of one strain but not in those of the other.

These results are derived from a study in which an impure material was tested. Studies on pharmaceutical grade material are now underway in a number of laboratories (IARC Information Bulletin No. 6).

The limited data available do not allow an evaluation of the carcinogenicity of disulfiram to be made.

Disulfiram can react with nitrite under mildly acid conditions, simulating those in the human stomach, to form *N*-nitrosodiethylamine, which has been shown to be carcinogenic in ten animal species (IARC, 1972).

4.2 Human data

No case reports or epidemiological studies were available to the Working Group.

5. References

ACGIH (American Conference of Government Industrial Hygienists) (1975) TLVs® Threshold Limit Values For Chemical Substances in Workroom Air Adopted by ACGIH for 1975, Cincinnati, Ohio, p. 38

Anon. (1973) Ethyl Tuads®, New York, R.T. Vanderbilt Co.

Anon. (1975) Materials and Compounding Ingredients for Rubber, New York, Bill Communications, pp. 37, 41, 48, 49, 56, 57

Anon. (1976) Alcoholism. Pharm. Index, 18, 11

Asmussen, E., Hald, J., Jacobsen, E. & Jørgensen, G. (1948a) Studies on the effect of tetraethylthiuram disulphide (Antabuse) and alcohol on respiration and circulation in normal human subjects. Acta pharmacol. toxicol. (Kbh.), 4, 297-304

Asmussen, E., Hald, J. & Larsen, V. (1948b) The pharmacological action of acetaldehyde on the human organism. Acta pharmacol. toxicol. (Kbh.), 4, 311-320

Bailey, G.C. (1931) Thiuram disulfides. US Patent 1,796,977, March 17, to Roessler & Hasslacher Chemical Co.

Brown, M.W., Porter, G.S. & Williams, A.E. (1974) The determination of disulfiram in blood, and of exhaled carbon disulphide using cathode ray polarography. J. Pharm. Pharmacol., 26, Suppl., 95P-96P

Child, G.P. & Crump, M. (1952) The toxicity of tetraethylthiuram disulphide (Antabuse) to mouse, rat, rabbit and dog. Acta pharmacol. toxicol. (Kbh.), 8, 305-314

Christensen, J. & Wase, A. (1954) Tetraethylthiuram disulphide and thyroid activity. Fed. Proc., 13, 343

Domar, G., Fredga, A. & Linderholm, H. (1949) A method for quantitative determination of tetraethylthiuram disulphide (Antabuse, Abstinyl) and its reduced form, diethyldithiocarbamic acid, as found in excreta. Acta chem. scand., 3, 1441-1442

Eldjarn, L. (1950a) The metabolism of tetraethyl thiuramdisulphide (Antabus, Aversan) in the rat, investigated by means of radioactive sulphur. Scand. J. clin. Lab. Invest., 2, 198-201

Eldjarn, L. (1950b) The metabolism of tetraethyl thiuramdisulphide (Antabus, Aversan) in man, investigated by means of radioactive sulphur. Scand. J. clin. Lab. Invest., 2, 202-208

Fishbein, L. & Zielinski, W.L., Jr (1967) Chromatography of carbamates. Chromat. Rev., 9, 37-101

Fitzhugh, O.G., Winter, W.J. & Nelson, A.A. (1952) Some observations on the chronic toxicity of antabuse (tetraethylthiuramdisulfide). Fed. Proc., 11, 345-346

Goldstein, M. (1966) Inhibition of norepinephrine biosynthesis at the dopamine-β-hydroxylation stage. Pharm. Rev., 18, 77-82

Grasselli, J.G., ed. (1973) Atlas of Spectral Data and Physical Constants for Organic Compounds, Cleveland, Ohio, Chemical Rubber Co., p. B-483

Grodzki, M. (1881) Concerning ethylated thioureas. Chem. Ber., 14, 2754-2758

Hald, J. & Jacobsen, E. (1948) The formation of acetaldehyde in the organism after ingestion of Antabuse (tetraethylthiuram disulphide) and alcohol. Acta pharmacol. toxicol. (Kbh.), 4, 305-310

Hald, J., Jacobsen, E. & Larsen, V. (1948) The sensitizing effect of tetraethylthiuramdisulphide (Antabuse) to ethyl alcohol. Acta pharmacol. toxicol. (Kbh.), 4, 285-296

Hald, J., Jacobsen, E. & Larsen, V. (1949) Formation of acetaldehyde in the organism in relation to dosage of Antabuse (tetraethylthiuram disulphide) and to alcohol-concentration in blood. Acta pharmacol. toxicol. (Kbh.), 5, 179-188

Holck, H.G.O., Lish, P.M., Sjogren, D.W., Westerfeld, W.W. & Malone, M.H. (1970) Effects of disulfiram on growth, longevity and reproduction of the albino rat. J. pharm. Sci., 59, 1267-1270

IARC (1972) IARC Monographs on the Evaluation of Carcinogenic Risk of Chemicals to Man, 1, Lyon, pp. 107-124

Innes, J.R.M., Ulland, B.M., Valerio, M.G., Petrucelli, L., Fishbein, L., Hart, E.R., Pallotta, A.J., Bates, R.R., Falk, H.L., Gart, J.J., Klein, M., Mitchell, I. & Peters, J. (1969) Bioassay of pesticides and industrial chemicals for tumorigenicity in mice: a preliminary note. J. nat. Cancer Inst., 42, 1101-1114

Johnston, C.D. & Prickett, C.S. (1952) The production of carbon disulfide from tetraethylthiuram disulfide (Antabuse) in rat liver. Biochim. biophys. acta, 9, 219-220

Kaslander, J. (1963) Formation of an S-glucuronide from tetraethylthiuram disulfide (Antabuse) in man. Biochim. biophys. acta, 71, 730-732

Larsen, V. (1948) The effect on experimental animals of Antabuse (tetraethylthiuramdisulphide) in combination with alcohol. Acta pharmacol. toxicol. (Kbh.), 4, 321-332

Lijinsky, W., Conrad, E. & Van de Bogart, R. (1972) Carcinogenic nitrosamines formed by drug/nitrite interactions. Nature (Lond.), 239,
165-167

Lilly, L.J. (1975) Investigations *in vitro* and *in vivo* of the effects of
disulfiram (Antabuse) on human lymphocyte chromosomes. Toxicology,
4, 331-340

van Logten, M.J. (1972) De Dithiocarbamaat-Alcohol-Reactie bij de Rat,
Terborg, The Netherlands, Bedrijf FA. Lammers

Merlevede, E. & Casier, H. (1961) Teneur en sulfure de carbone de l'air
expiré chez des personnes normales ou sous l'influence de l'alcool
éthylique au cours du traitement par l'Antabuse (disulfiram) et le
diéthyldithiocarbamate de soude. Arch. int. Pharmacodyn., 132,
427-453

Neims, A.H., Coffey, D.S. & Hellerman, L. (1966) Interaction between
tetraethylthiuram disulfide and the sulfhydryl groups of D-amino acid
oxidase and of hemoglobin. J. biol. Chem., 241, 5941-5948

NTIS (National Technical Information Service) (1968) Evaluation of Carcino-
genic, Teratogenic and Mutagenic Activities of Selected Pesticides and
Industrial Chemicals, Vol. 1, Carcinogenic Study, Washington DC, US
Department of Commerce

Nygaard, A.P. & Sumner, J.B. (1952) D-Glyceraldehyde 3-phosphate dehydrogenase; a comparison with liver aldehyde dehydrogenase. Arch. Biochem.
Biophys., 39, 119-128

Porter, G.S. & Williams, A. (1972) The determination of low concentrations
of disulfiram by cathode ray polarography. J. Pharm. Pharmacol., 24,
Suppl., 144P-145P

Prickett, C.S. & Johnston, C.D. (1953) The *in vivo* production of carbon
disulfide from tetraethylthiuramdisulfide (Antabuse). Biochim.
biophys. acta, 12, 542-546

Richert, D.A., Vanderline, R. & Westerfeld, W.W. (1950) The composition
of rat liver xanthine oxidase and its inhibition by antabuse. J. biol.
Chem., 186, 261-274

Schmähl, D., Krüger, F.W., Ivankovic, S. & Preissler, P. (1971) Verminderung
der Toxizität von Dimethylnitrosamin bei Ratten und Mäusen nach Behandlung mit Disulfiram. Arzneimittel Forsch., 21, 1560-1562

Schmähl, D., Krüger, F.W., Habs, M. & Diehl, B. (1976) Influence of disulfiram
on the organotropy of the carcinogenic effect of dimethylnitrosamine and
diethylnitrosamine in rats. Z. Krebsforsch., 85, 271-276

94

Shaver, F.W. (1968) Rubber chemicals. In: Kirk, R.E. & Othmer, D.F., eds, Encyclopedia of Chemical Technology, 2nd ed., Vol. 17, New York, John Wiley & Sons, pp. 509-514

Stecher, P.G., ed. (1968) The Merck Index, 8th ed., Rahway, NJ, Merck & Co., p. 393

Strömme, J.H. (1963) Inhibition of hexokinase by disulfiram and diethyl-dithiocarbamate. Biochem. Pharmacol., 12, 157-166

Strömme, J.H. (1965) Metabolism of disulfiram and diethyldithiocarbamate in rats with demonstration of an in vivo ethanol-induced inhibition of the glucuronic acid conjugation of the thiol. Biochem. Pharmacol., 14, 393-410

US International Trade Commission (1975) Synthetic Organic Chemicals, US Production and Sales of Rubber-Processing Chemicals, 1974 Preliminary, Washington DC, US Government Printing Office, p. 8

US Tariff Commission (1941) Synthetic Organic Chemicals, US Production and Sales, 1940, Report No. 148, Second Series, Washington DC, US Government Printing Office, p. 50

Wattenberg, L.W. (1974) Inhibition of carcinogenic and toxic effects of polycyclic hydrocarbons by several sulfur-containing compounds. J. nat. Cancer Inst., 52, 1583-1587

Wattenberg, L.W. (1975) Inhibition of dimethylhydrazine-induced neoplasia of the large intestine by disulfiram. J. nat. Cancer Inst., 54, 1005-1006

Weast, R.C., ed. (1975) CRC Handbook of Chemistry and Physics, 56th ed., Cleveland, Ohio, Chemical Rubber Co., p. C-272

Wells, J. & Koves, E. (1974) Detection of carbon disulphide (a disulfiram metabolite) in expired air by gas chromatography. J. Chromat., 92, 442-444

Zemaitis, M.A. & Greene, F.E. (1976) Impairment of hepatic microsomal drug metabolism in the rat during daily disulfiram administration. Biochem. Pharmacol., 25, 1355-1360

DULCIN

1. Chemical and Physical Data

1.1 Synonyms and trade names

Chem. Abstr. Reg. Serial No.: 150-69-6

Chem. Abstr. Name: (4-Ethoxyphenyl) urea

para-Ethoxyphenylurea; *para*-phenetolcarbamide; *para*-phenetolecarbamide; *para*-phenetylurea

Dulcine; Sucrol; Valzin

1.2 Chemical formula and molecular weight

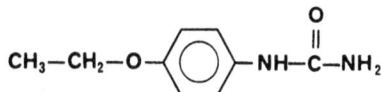

$$CH_3-CH_2-O-\underset{}{\bigcirc}-NH-\overset{\overset{\textstyle O}{\|}}{C}-NH_2$$

$C_9H_{12}N_2O_2$ Mol. wt: 180.2

1.3 Chemical and physical properties of the substance

(a) <u>Description</u>: Needles (Stecher, 1968)

(b) <u>Melting-point</u>: 173-174°C (Weast, 1975)

(c) <u>Spectroscopy data</u>: λ_{max} 290 nm and 242 nm in ethanol (E_1^1 = 110 and 1001) (Weast, 1975); for infra-red spectra, see Grasselli (1973).

(d) <u>Solubility</u>: 1 part soluble in 800 parts of cold water, 50 parts of hot water or 25 parts of ethanol (Stecher, 1968)

(e) <u>Stability</u>: Partially decomposes on heating with water; hydrolyses in 0.1 N acetic acid (Richter, 1950)

1.4 Technical products and impurities

No data were available to the Working Group.

2. Production, Use, Occurrence and Analysis

For important background information on this section, see preamble, p. 15.

2.1 Production and use

The preparation of dulcin was first reported in 1883 by Berlinerblau, who synthesized it by reacting *para*-phenetidine with phosgene and ammonia (Stecher, 1968).

Dulcin can be prepared by: (<u>a</u>) reacting *para*-phenetidine hydrochloride with urea; (<u>b</u>) heating *para*-ethoxyphenylurethan and ammonia; (<u>c</u>) treating ammonium *para*-ethoxyphenyldithiocarbamate with lead carbamate; (<u>d</u>) ethylating *para*-hydroxyphenylurea; (<u>e</u>) heating di(*para*-ethoxyphenyl)urea with urea, ammonium carbamate and ammonium carbonate; or (<u>f</u>) reacting ammonia with *para*-ethoxyphenyl isocyanate (Kurzer, 1963).

Commercial production of dulcin was reported in the US between 1944 (US Tariff Commission, 1946) and 1955 (US Tariff Commission, 1956). No indication has been found that it is currently being produced in commercial quantities in the US, although two companies produce it for research purposes.

Dulcin is 250 times as sweet as sucrose, has a taste preferable to that of saccharin and when used in combination with saccharin has a synergistic sweetening effect and enhances the sugar-like flavour (Weinberg, 1964). The only known use of dulcin was as a non-nutritive sweetener (Stecher, 1968), but it has not been used as such in the US for over 20 years since it is not approved by the Food and Drug Administration (Sanders, 1953).

In 1967, the Joint FAO/WHO Expert Committee on Food Additives recommended that dulcin should not be used as a food additive (WHO, 1968). In Japan, the use of dulcin as a food additive was forbidden in 1968 (Japanese Union of Food Additives Associations, 1974).

2.2 Occurrence

Dulcin is not known to occur as a natural product.

2.3 Analysis

Numerous methods have been described for the separation and identification of artificial sweetening agents by thin-layer chromatography on different substrates and using a variety of reagents for their detection.

Dulcin has been determined by thin-layer chromatography in carbonated drinks and fruit juices, with limits of detection of 5 and 7 mg/kg, respectively (de la Torre Boronat & Ribalta, 1972); in a variety of soft drinks, with a limit of detection of 0.03% (Korbelak, 1969); and in some Japanese foods, with a limit of detection of 1-8 μg/ml (Uchiyama *et al.*, 1969). A detailed method for its determination in food products, with a detection limit ranging from 0.01-2 μg depending on the chromogenic spray reagent employed, includes a preliminary column chromatography clean-up (Takeshita, 1972). A comparison has been made of the sensitivity of different spray reagents on different thin-layer chromatography substrates, with detection limits for dulcin ranging from 0.1-1.0 μg (Nagasawa *et al.*, 1970). Paper chromatography has been used for its detection in foods, with a limit of 12.5 μg (Matsumoto, 1969), and in wine (Rotolo, 1972).

Gas chromatography has been employed to separate the methylated derivative of dulcin from other sweeteners (König, 1971).

3. Biological Data Relevant to the Evaluation of Carcinogenic Risk to Man

3.1 Carcinogenicity and related studies in animals

(a) Oral administration

Rat: Groups of 10 male and 10 female 4-week old Osborne-Mendel rats were fed diets containing 0, 0.01, 0.1, 0.25, 0.5 or 1% dulcin for up to 2 years; 25% of the animals receiving 1% dulcin died within one year. Ten animals receiving 1% in the diet, 2 receiving 0.5% and 1 receiving 0.1% developed hepatic-cell adenomas, some of which were described as 'histologically malignant'. No such tumours occurred in rats fed 0.01% dulcin or in those of the control group (Fitzhugh *et al.*, 1951).

Groups of 10-25 male rats (strain not specified) were fed diets containing 0, 0.001, 0.01, 0.1, 0.5 or 1% dulcin for 2 years. After 18 months, 7/10, 7/10, 7/10, 8/20, 7/20 and 4/25 rats in the respective groups were still alive; no liver tumours were observed (Ikeda et al., 1960).

A group of 30 14-week old rats (mainly male, strain not specified) was fed 20 g of a diet containing 1% commercial dulcin (m.p. 169-170°C) daily for up to 24 months. Thirty rats fed the basal diet alone served as controls. All of 30 rats which received a diet containing 0.1% butter yellow and served as positive controls died with liver tumours within 21-24 months. After one year, 26 dulcin-treated rats and 26 controls were alive; by the end of the experiment, 9 treated and 13 control rats were still alive. Papillomas of the pelvic epithelium and of the bladder occurred in about 75% of 23 treated animals and in none of 19 controls. Stones were present in the renal pelvis and bladder of about 66% of the 23 treated animals. All stones were associated with papillomas, but the papillomas did not always occur in the area of the urinary tract where the stone was located (Bär & Griepentrog, 1958; Griepentrog, 1959).

A group of 80 white rats (sex unspecified) received different doses of dulcin for lifespan. Fifteen rats receiving 0.2 g/kg bw/day survived 12 months, and the last rat survived 22 months; no carcinogenic effect was seen (Lettré & Wrba, 1955).

(b) Other experimental systems

Pre- and postnatal exposures: A group of 20 male and 30 female rats was given oral intubations of 0.2 g/kg bw/day dulcin in Tween-methyl cellulose solution for 400 days (total dose, 17 g), at which time 60% of the animals were still alive. Half of these animals received no dulcin from then on and were observed until death; the remaining animals continued to receive the dulcin treatment, and total doses of up to 33 g/animal were given. No malignant tumours were reported. Of 30 controls given the Tween-methyl cellulose vehicle alone, one developed a fibroadenoma. During the experiment an unstated number of treated males and 20 treated females were mated; the 39 male offspring were treated at 8 weeks of age with 0.2 g/kg bw/day for 660 days (total dose, 29 g), at which time the 5 survivors were killed. No malignant tumours were reported (Bekemeier et al., 1958).

3.2 Other relevant biological data

(a) Experimental systems

The oral LD_{50}'s for dulcin in young and adult rats are 4.9 and 3.2 g/kg bw, respectively (Bekemeier et al., 1958). Doses of about 0.5 g/kg bw dulcin per day were lethal to rats within several days to a few weeks (Bekemeier et al., 1958; Lettré & Wrba, 1955).

After its oral administration to rats, dulcin is absorbed rapidly (Akagi et al., 1965; Kojima et al., 1966) and is distributed throughout the body, with highest concentrations in the liver, kidneys, brain and lungs; tissue levels diminished to one-tenth within 24 hours after dosing (Akagi et al., 1965).

Akagi et al. (1966) found that 3% of a dose of dulcin was excreted unchanged in the urine of treated rabbits, 27% was excreted as dulcin N-glucuronide, a further 40% was excreted collectively as para-hydroxyphenylurea and its O-sulphate and O-glucuronide, and there were small amounts of urinary para-aminophenol.

No deleterious effects were seen on the 18th day of gestation in the foetuses of female mice given 10-50 mg/kg bw dulcin intragastrically on days 8-10 of pregnancy. Retarded growth and some deaths were observed among the progeny of dams treated on days 6-7 of pregnancy (Tanaka, 1964).

Dulcin reacts with nitrite to form N-nitrosodulcin (Mirvish, 1975).

(b) Man

Thorough studies on human volunteers, including several diabetics, showed that the ingestion of 0.1-0.6 g dulcin/day for one year produced no adverse effects (Rost & Braun, 1926).

Two deaths in children have been associated with the ingestion of 8-10 g dulcin. In adults, doses of 20-40 g dulcin produced dizziness, nausea, methaemoglobinaemia with cyanosis, hypotension and, in one case, coronary disturbance (Buhr, 1948).

3.3 Case reports and epidemiological studies

No data were available to the Working Group.

4. Comments on Data Reported and Evaluation

4.1 Animal data

Dulcin has been tested only in rats by oral administration. Increased incidences of liver-cell adenomas were observed in one study, and papillomas of the renal pelvis and bladder, associated with stone formation, were seen in another study, but these results were not confirmed in two other trials. No evaluation of the carcinogenicity of dulcin can be made.

4.2 Human data

No case reports or epidemiological studies were available to the Working Group.

5. References

Akagi, M., Oketani, Y. & Uematsu, T. (1965) Studies on food additives. IX. Estimation of *p*-ethoxyphenylurea in biological materials and physiological disposition in the animals. Chem. pharm. Bull., 13, 1200-1206

Akagi, M., Aoki, I. & Uematsu, T. (1966) Studies on food additives. X. The metabolism of *p*-ethoxyphenylurea in the rabbit. Chem. pharm. Bull., 14, 1-9

Bär, F. & Griepentrog, F. (1958) Zur chronischen Toxizität von Dulcin (*p*-Äthoxyphenylharnstoff). Naturwissenschaften, 45, 390-391

Bekemeier, H., Hannig, E. & Pfennigsdorf, G. (1958) Zur Kenntnis von Verträglichkeit und Cancerogenität des *p*-Äthoxy-phenylharnstoffes. Arzneimittel-Forsch., 8, 150-151

Buhr, G. (1948) Vier Vergiftungsfälle mit dem Süssstoff Dulcin (*para*-Phenetolcarbamid). Med. Klinik, 43, 105-108

Fitzhugh, O.G., Nelson, A.A. & Frawley, J.P. (1951) A comparison of the chronic toxicities of synthetic sweetening agents. J. Amer. pharm. Ass., 40, 583-586

Grasselli, J.G., ed. (1973) Atlas of Spectral Data and Physical Constants for Organic Compounds, Cleveland, Ohio, Chemical Rubber Co., p. B-985

Griepentrog, F. (1959) Tumoren der Harnwege und Harnsteine in chronischen Versuchen mit dem Süssstoff *p*-Phenetylcarbamid. Arzneimittel Forsch., 9, 123-125

Ikeda, Y., Omori, Y., Oka, S., Shinoda, M. & Tsuzi, K. (1960) Studies on chronic toxicity of dulcin. J. Fd Hyg. Soc. Japan, 1, 62-69

Japanese Union of Food Additives Associations (1974) The Japanese Standards of Food Additives, 3rd ed., Tokyo, pp. 11-12

Kojima, S., Ichibagase, H. & Iguchi, S. (1966) Studies on synthetic sweetening agents. VII. Absorption and excretion of sodium cyclamate. Chem. pharm. Bull., 14, 965-971

König, H. (1971) Trennung, Nachweis und Bestimmung der künstlichen Süssstoffe Cyclamat, Dulcin und Saccharin mittels Gas-Chromatographie. Z. analyt. Chem., 255, 123-125

Korbelak, T. (1969) TLC identification of four artificial sweeteners in beverages: collaborative study. J. Ass. off. analyt. Chem., 52, 487-491

Kurzer, F. (1963) Arylureas. In: Rabjohn, N., ed., Organic Syntheses, Vol. 4, New York, John Wiley & Sons, pp. 52-54

Lettré, H. & Wrba, H. (1955) Die Wirkung des Süssstoffes Dulcin bei langdauernder Fütterung. Naturwissenschaften, 42, 217

Matsumoto, S. (1969) Color reactions of sweeteners. Tokyo Toritsu Eisei Kenkyusho Kenkyu Nempo, 21, 89-92

Mirvish, S.S. (1975) Formation of N-nitroso compounds. Chemistry, kinetics and in vivo occurrence. Toxicol. appl. Pharmacol., 31, 325-351

Nagasawa, K., Yoshidome, H. & Anryu, K. (1970) Separation and detection of synthetic sweeteners by thin-layer chromatography. J. Chromat., 52, 173-176

Richter, F., ed. (1950) Beilsteins Handbuch der organischen Chemie, 4th ed., Vol. 13, Syst. No. 1848, pp. 253-254

Rost, E. & Braun, A. (1926) Zur Pharmakologie des para-Phenetolcarbamids, Dulcin. Arb. Reichsgesundh. Amte, 57, 212-220

Rotolo, A. (1972) Identificazione di alcuni edulcoranti sintetici nei vini. Riv. Viticol. Enol., 25, 301-310

Sanders, H.J. (1953) Sweet but noncaloric. Industr. Eng. Chem., 45, 11A, 13A

Stecher, P.G. ed. (1968) The Merck Index, 8th ed., Rahway, NJ, Merck & Co., pp. 399-400

Takeshita, R. (1972) Application of column and thin-layer chromatography to the detection of artificial sweeteners in foods. J. Chromat., 66, 283-293

Tanaka, R. (1964) The toxicity of synthetic sweetening agents to mice embryo. Japan. J. Publ. Hlth, 11, 909-915

de la Torre Boronat, C. & Ribalta, C. (1972) Investigación de edulcorantes en bebidas del mercado, aromáticas y no alcohólicas. Circ. Farm., 30, 231-242

Uchiyama, S., Kondo, T. & Kawashiro, I. (1969) A new fluorometric analysis of dulcin using sodium nitrite. I. Establishment of quantitative method and its application to food analysis. Yakugaku Zasshi, 89, 828-832

US Tariff Commission (1946) Synthetic Organic Chemicals, US Production and Sales, 1944, Report No. 155, Second Series, Washington DC, US Government Printing Office, p. 99

US Tariff Commission (1956) Synthetic Organic Chemicals, US Production and Sales, 1955, Report No. 198, Second Series, Washington DC, US Government Printing Office, p. 117

Weast, R.C., ed. (1975) CRC Handbook of Chemistry and Physics, 56th ed., Cleveland, Ohio, Chemical Rubber Co., p. C-532

Weinberg, B. (1964) Sweetening chemicals challenge sucrose. Canad. Chem. Processing, April, 77, 80

WHO (1968) Specifications for the identity and purity of food additives and their toxicological evaluation: some flavouring substances and non-nutritive sweetening agents. Wld Hlth Org. techn. Rep. Ser., No. 383, pp. 100-103

ETHYL SELENAC

1. Chemical and Physical Data

1.1 Synonyms and trade names

Chem. Abstr. Reg. Serial No.: 12367-47-4

Chem. Abstr. Name: Tetrakis(diethylcarbamodithioato-S,S')selenium

Selenium diethyldithiocarbamate, tetrakis(diethyldithiocarbamato)-selenium

Ethyl seleram

1.2 Chemical formula and molecular weight

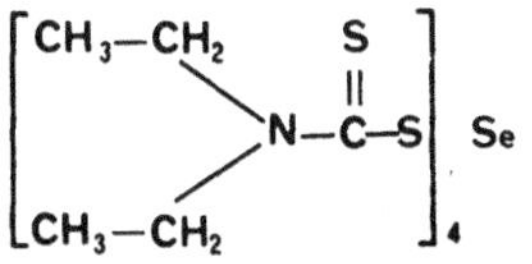

$$\left[\begin{array}{c} CH_3-CH_2 \\ \\ CH_3-CH_2 \end{array} \right\rangle N-\overset{\overset{\textstyle S}{\|}}{C}-S \right]_4 Se$$

$C_{20}H_{40}N_4S_8Se$ Mol. wt: 672.0

1.3 Chemical and physical properties of the pure substance

No data were available to the Working Group.

1.4 Technical products and impurities

Ethyl selenac is available commercially in the US with the following typical specifications: yellow powder; density, 1.32 ± 0.03; melting range, 59-85°C; moisture (at 40-45°C), 2.5% max.; ash, 0.5% max.; particle size, 99.5% passes through a 100-mesh screen; selenium content, 10.5-12.7% (Anon., 1974, 1975). The chemical is also available in a dispersion containing 70% ethyl selenac and 30% ethylene-propylene-diene binder (Anon. 1975).

2. Production, Use, Occurrence and Analysis

For important background information on this section, see preamble, p. 15.

2.1 Production and use

The usual method for the preparation of water-insoluble dialkyldithio-carbamate metal salts is precipitation of the metal salt from an aqueous preparation of the sodium dialkyldithiocarbamate (Shaver, 1968).

Commercial production of ethyl selenac was first reported in the US in 1938 (US Tariff Commission, 1939); only one manufacturer reported production in 1974 (US International Trade Commission, 1975). It is estimated that less than 1 million kg are produced annually in France.

Ethyl selenac is used in the rubber-processing industry as an accelerator to produce desired physical properties in vulcanized rubber in a shorter curing time and at lower sulphur levels than with conventional accelerators (Supp & Gibbs, 1974). It is used in compounding natural, butadiene, isobutylene-isoprene and styrene-butadiene rubbers. It is an effective accelerator for low-sulphur and sulphur-less heat-resistant compounds, does not cause discolouration and is generally used with thiazoles to balance scorch and cure characteristics (Anon., 1975).

According to the US Occupational Safety and Health Administration health standards for air contaminants, an employee's exposure to selenium compounds should not exceed 0.2 mg/m^3 (as Se) in the workplace air during any eight-hour workshift for a forty-hour work week (US Code of Federal Regulations, 1975). In the USSR, the maximum allowable concentration of selenium compounds in the work environment is 0.1 mg/m^3 (Winell, 1975).

2.2 Occurrence

Ethyl selenac is not known to occur as a natural product.

2.3 Analysis

Methods for the determination of selenium by gas chromatography have been reviewed (Young & Christian, 1973). Gas chromatography coupled with a microwave-emission spectrometric detection system has been used for determination of trace amounts of selenium in environmental samples (Talmi & Andren, 1974). Ethyl selenac has been determined in rubber additives by both atomic absorption spectrometry and wet analytical determination of selenium (Supp & Gibbs, 1974).

Methods for the chromatographic analysis of carbamates, including thiocarbamates, have been reviewed (Fishbein & Zielinski, 1967). A thin-layer chromatographic-spectrophotofluorimetric method (van Hoof & Heyndrickx, 1973) is suitable for the analysis of a variety of metal dithiocarbamates, although it was not applied to ethyl selenac itself.

3. Biological Data Relevant to the Evaluation of Carcinogenic Risk to Man[1]

3.1 Carcinogenicity and related studies in animals

(a) Oral administration

Mouse: Groups of 18 male and 18 female (C57BL/6xC3H/Anf)F_1 mice and 18 male and 18 female C57BL/6xAKR)F_1 mice received commercial ethyl selenac (m.p. 59-85°C) according to the following schedule: 10 mg/kg bw in gelatine at 7 days of age by stomach tube and the same amount (not adjusted for increasing body weight) daily up to 4 weeks of age; subsequently, the mice were given 26 mg ethyl selenac per kg of diet. The dose was the maximum tolerated dose for infant and young mice but not necessarily so for adults. The experiment was terminated when the animals were about 78 weeks of age, at which time 16, 14, 17 and 14 mice in the four groups, respectively, were still alive. Tumour incidences were compared with those in 79-90 necropsied mice of each sex and strain, which either had been untreated or had received gelatine only. Tumours occurred in 16/18 necropsied males (12 hepatomas, 3 reticulum-cell sarcomas and 1 sebaceous-gland carcinoma) of the first strain and

---

[1]See also the monograph on selenium and selenium compounds (IARC, 1975).

in 5/17 males (3 hepatomas, 1 reticulum-cell sarcoma and 3 pulmonary tumours) and 4/17 females (3 reticulum-cell sarcomas and 1 pulmonary tumour) of the second strain. The increased incidence of hepatomas in (C57BL/6x C3H/Anf)F$_1$ males over that in controls (12/18 compared with 8/79) was significant (P<0.001) (Innes *et al.*, 1969; NTIS, 1968).

(b) Subcutaneous administration

Mouse: Groups of 18 male and 18 female (C57BL/6xC3H/Anf)F$_1$ mice and 18 male and 18 female (C57BL/6xAKR)F$_1$ mice were given single s.c. injections of 464 mg/kg bw ethyl selenac (m.p. 59-85°C) in 0.5% gelatine on the 28th day of life and were observed until they were about 78 weeks of age, at which time 13, 17, 18 and 18 mice in the four groups, respectively, were still alive. Tumour incidences were compared with those in groups of 141, 154, 161 and 157 untreated or vehicle-injected controls that were necropsied. Incidences were not increased (P>0.05) for any tumour type in any sex-strain subgroup or in the combined sexes of either strain (NTIS, 1968) [The Working Group noted that a negative result obtained with a single s.c. injection may not be an adequate basis for discounting carcinogenicity].

3.2 Other relevant biological data

No data were available to the Working Group.

3.3 Case reports and epidemiological studies

No data were available to the Working Group.

4. Comments on Data Reported and Evaluation

4.1 Animal data

Ethyl selenac has been tested by oral administration and by single subcutaneous injection in two strains of mice. It produced an increased incidence of liver-cell tumours in males of one strain but did not significantly increase the incidence of tumours in the other. The available data are insufficient to allow an evaluation of the carcinogenicity of this compound to be made.

4.2 Human data

No case reports or epidemiological studies were available to the Working Group.

5.   References

Anon. (1974)   Ethyl Selenac Ⓡ, Norwalk, Connecticut, R.T. Vanderbilt Co.

Anon. (1975)   Materials and Compounding Ingredients for Rubber, New York, Bill Communications, pp. 51, 53

Fishbein, L. & Zielinski, W.L., Jr (1967)   Chromatography of carbamates. Chromat. Rev., 9, 37-101

van Hoof, F. & Heyndrickx, A. (1973)   Thin layer chromatographic-spectro-photophuorimetric methods for the determination of dithio- and thiol-carbamates after hydrolysis and coupling with NBD-Cl. Ghent. Rijks-univ. Fac. Landbl. Med., 38, 911-916

IARC (1975)   IARC Monographs on the Evaluation of Carcinogenic Risk of Chemicals to Man, 9, Some Aziridines, N-, S- and O-Mustards and Selenium, Lyon, pp. 250-251

Innes, J.R.M., Ulland, B.M., Valerio, M.G., Petrucelli, L., Fishbein, L., Hart, E.R., Pallotta, A.J., Bates, R.R., Falk, H.L., Gart, J.J., Klein, M., Mitchell, I. & Peters, J. (1969)   Bioassay of pesticides and industrial chemicals for tumorigenicity in mice: a preliminary note. J. nat. Cancer Inst., 42, 1101-1114

NTIS (National Technical Information Service) (1968)   Evaluation of Carcinogenic, Teratogenic and Mutagenic Activities of Selected Pesticides and Industrial Chemicals, Vol. 1, Carcinogenic Study, Washington DC, US Department of Commerce

Shaver, F.W. (1968)   Rubber chemicals. In: Kirk, R.E. & Othmer, D.F., eds, Encyclopedia of Chemical Technology, 2nd ed., Vol. 17, New York, John Wiley & Sons, p. 513

Supp, G.R. & Gibbs, I. (1974)   The determination of selenium and tellurium in organic accelerators used in the vulcanization process for natural and synthetic rubbers by atomic absorption spectrometry. Atomic Absorption Newslett., 13, 71-73

Talmi, Y. & Andren, A.W. (1974)   Determination of selenium in environmental samples using gas chromatography with a microwave emission spectrometric detection system. Analyt. Chem., 46, 2122-2126

US Code of Federal Regulations (1975)   Air Contaminants, Title 29, part. 1910.1000, Washington DC, US Government Printing Office, p. 61

US International Trade Commission (1975)   Synthetic Organic Chemicals, US Production and Sales of Rubber-Processing Chemicals, 1974 Preliminary, Washington DC, US Government Printing Office, p. 7

US Tariff Commission (1939) Synthetic Organic Chemicals, US Production and Sales, 1938, Report No. 136, Second Series, Washington DC, US Government Printing Office, p. 45

Winell, M.A. (1975) An international comparison of hygienic standards for chemicals in the work environment. Ambio, 4, 34-36

Young, J.W. & Christian G.D. (1973) Gas-chromatographic determination of selenium. Analyt. chim. acta., 65, 127-138

ETHYL TELLURAC

1. Chemical and Physical Data

1.1 Synonyms and trade names

Chem. Abstr. Reg. Serial No.: 12367-49-6

Chem. Abstr. Name: Tetrakis(diethylcarbamodithioato-S,S')tellurium

Tellurium diethyldithiocarbamate

1.2 Chemical formula and molecular weight

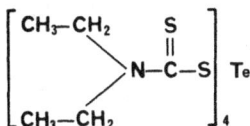

$$\left[\begin{array}{c} CH_3-CH_2 \\ \\ \\ CH_3-CH_2 \end{array} \hspace{-1em} \begin{array}{c} \\ \diagdown \\ \diagup \\ \end{array} N-\overset{\overset{\textstyle S}{\|}}{C}-S \right]_4 Te$$

$$C_{20}H_{40}N_4S_8Te \qquad \text{Mol. wt: } 720.6$$

1.3 Chemical and physical properties of the pure substance

No data were available to the Working Group.

1.4 Technical products and impurities

Ethyl tellurac is available commercially in the US with the following typical specifications: orange-yellow powder; density, 1.44 ± 0.03; melting range, 108-118°C; particle size, 100% passes through a 30-mesh screen; ash, 2.5% max.; tellurium content, 17.5-19.5%; heating loss, 1.0% max. (Anon., 1968). For rubber processing, ethyl tellurac is available in rod form containing 80% of active ingredient and in a dispersion containing 25% of a binder (Anon., 1975).

2. Production, Use, Occurrence and Analysis

For important background information on this section, see preamble, p. 15.

2.1 Production and use

Ethyl tellurac can be prepared by the addition of carbon disulphide to an aqueous solution of diethylamine and sodium hydroxide (Shaver, 1968), followed by reaction of the resulting sodium diethyldithiocarbamate with potassium tellurite (Husebye & Svaeren, 1973).

Commercial production of ethyl tellurac was first reported in the US in 1939 (US Tariff Commission, 1940); only one US manufacturer reported production in 1974 (US International Trade Commission, 1975). Less than 1 million kg are produced annually in the Benelux countries and in France.

Ethyl tellurac is used in the rubber-processing industry as an accelerator in compounding natural, styrene-butadiene, nitrile-butadiene, ethylene-propylene diene and isobutylene-isoprene rubbers. It produces high-modulus vulcanization and is generally used with thiazole modifiers (Anon., 1975).

2.2 Occurrence

Ethyl tellurac is not known to occur as natural product.

2.3 Analysis

Ethyl tellurac in rubber additives can be determined by atomic absorption spectrometric or gravimetric determination of tellurium (Supp & Gibbs, 1974).

Methods for the chromatographic analysis of carbamates, including thiocarbamates, have been reviewed (Fishbein & Zielinski, 1967). A thin-layer chromatographic-spectrophotofluorimetric method (van Hoof & Heyndrickx, 1973) is suitable for the analysis of a variety of metal dithiocarbamates, although it was not applied to ethyl tellurac itself.

3. Biological Data Relevant to the Evaluation of Carcinogenic Risk to Man

3.1 Carcinogenicity and related studies in animals

(a) Oral administration

Mouse: Groups of 18 male and 18 female (C57BL/6xC3H/Anf)F$_1$ mice and

116

18 male and 18 female (C57BL/6xAKR)F$_1$ mice received commercial ethyl tellurac (m.p. 108-118°C) according to the following schedule: 46.4 mg/kg bw in gelatine at 7 days of age by stomach tube and the same amount (not adjusted for increasing body weight) daily up to 4 weeks of age; subsequently, the mice were given 149 mg ethyl tellurac per kg of diet. The dose was the maximum tolerated dose for infant and young mice but not necessarily so for adults. The experiment was terminated when the animals were about 78 weeks of age, at which time 15 males and 18 females of each strain were still alive. Tumour incidences were compared with those in 79-90 necropsied mice of each sex and strain, which either had been untreated or had received gelatine only. Tumours developed in 9/16 necropsied males and in 2/18 necropsied females of the first strain and in 6/18 necropsied males and 6/18 necropsied females of the second strain. Hepatomas occurred in 4/16 males of the first strain and in 3/18 males of the second strain, compared with 8/79 and 5/90 in controls (P>0.05 for each strain). The incidence of lung tumours in males and females of the second strain was 7/36, compared with 12/172 in controls [P<0.02] (Innes *et al.*, 1969; NTIS, 1968).

(b) Subcutaneous administration

Mouse: Groups of 18 male and 18 female (C57BL/6xC3H/Anf)F$_1$ mice and 18 male and 18 female (C57BL/6xAKR)F$_1$ mice were given single s.c. injections of 1000 mg/kg bw ethyl tellurac (m.p. 108-118°C) in 0.5% gelatine on the 28th day of life and were observed until they were about 78 weeks of age, at which time 14, 17, 17 and 15 mice in the four groups, respectively, were still alive. Tumour incidences were compared with those in groups of 141, 154, 161 and 157 untreated or vehicle-injected controls that were necropsied. Incidences were not increased (P>0.05) for any tumour type in any sex-strain subgroup or in the combined sexes of either strain (NTIS, 1968) [The Working Group noted that a negative result obtained with a single s.c. injection may not be an adequate basis for discounting carcinogenicity].

3.2 Other relevant biological data

No data were available to the Working Group.

3.3 Case reports and epidemiological studies

No data were available to the Working Group.

4. Comments on Data Reported and Evaluation

4.1 Animal data

Ethyl tellurac has been tested by oral administration and by single subcutaneous injection in two strains of mice. There was a small but significant increase in the number of lung tumours in males and females of one strain combined after its oral administration. The available data are insufficient to allow an evaluation of the carcinogenicity of this compound.

4.2 Human data

No case reports or epidemiological studies were available to the Working Group.

5. References

Anon. (1968) Ethyl Tellurac ®, New York, R.T. Vanderbilt Co.

Anon. (1975) Materials and Compounding Ingredients for Rubber, New York, Bill Communications, pp. 47, 51, 54

Fishbein, L. & Zielinski, W.L., Jr (1967) Chromatography of carbamates. Chromat. Rev., 9, 37-101

van Hoof, F. & Heyndrickx, A. (1973) Thin layer chromatographic-spectrophotophuorimetric methods for the determination of dithio- and thiolcarbamates after hydrolysis and coupling with NBD-Cl. Ghent. Rijksuniv. Fac. Landbl. Med., 38, 911-916

Husebye, S. & Svaeren, S.E. (1973) The crystal and molecular structure of tetrakis(diethyldithiocarbamato)tellurium (IV). Acta chem. scand., 27, 763-778

Innes, J.R.M., Ulland, B.M., Valerio, M.G., Petrucelli, L., Fishbein, L., Hart, E.R., Pallotta, A.J., Bates, R.R., Falk, H.L., Gart, J.J., Klein, M., Mitchell, I. & Peters, J. (1969) Bioassay of pesticides and industrial chemicals for tumorigenicity in mice: a preliminary note. J. nat. Cancer Inst., 42, 1101-1114

NTIS (National Technical Information Service) (1968) Evaluation of Carcinogenic, Teratogenic and Mutagenic Activities of Selected Pesticides and Industrial Chemicals, Vol. 1, Carcinogenic Study, Washington DC, US Department of Commerce

Shaver, F.W. (1968) Rubber chemicals. In: Kirk, R.E. & Othmer, D.F., eds, Encyclopedia of Chemical Technology, 2nd ed., Vol. 17, New York, John Wiley & Sons, p. 513

Supp, G.R. & Gibbs, I. (1974) The determination of selenium and tellurium in organic accelerators used in the vulcanization process for natural and synthetic rubbers by atomic absorption spectrometry. Atomic Absorption Newslett., 13, 71-73

US International Trade Commission (1975) Synthetic Organic Chemicals, US Production and Sales of Rubber-Processing Chemicals, 1974 Preliminary, Washington DC, US Government Printing Office, p. 7

US Tariff Commission (1940) Synthetic Organic Chemicals, US Production and Sales, 1939, Report No. 140, Second Series, Washington DC, US Government Printing Office, p. 45

FERBAM

1. Chemical and Physical Data

1.1 Synonyms and trade names

Chem. Abstr. Reg. Serial No.: 14484-64-1

Chem. Abstr. Name: Tris(dimethylcarbamodithioato-S,S')iron

Dimethylcarbamodithioic acid, iron complex; dimethylcarbamodithioic acid, iron (3+) salt; dimethyldithiocarbamic acid, iron salt; dimethyldithiocarbamic acid, iron (3+) salt; ferric dimethyldithio-carbamate; iron dimethyldithiocarbamate; tris(dimethyldithiocarbamato)-iron; tris(N,N-dimethyldithiocarbamato) iron (III)

Aafertis; Bercema Fertam 50; Ferbam 50; Ferbam, iron salt; Ferbeck; Fermate; Fermate Ferbam fungicide; Ferradow; Fuklasin Ultra; Hexaferb; Karbam Black; Stauffer ferbam; Sup'r Flo Ferbam Flowable; Trifungol; Vancide FE-95

1.2 Chemical formula and molecular weight

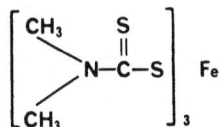

$$\left[\begin{array}{c} CH_3 \\ \diagdown \\ N-C-S \\ \diagup \quad \| \\ CH_3 \quad S \end{array} \right]_3 Fe$$

$C_9H_{18}FeN_3S_6$ Mol. wt: 416.5

1.3 Chemical and physical properties of the substance

From Stecher (1968), unless otherwise specified

(a) Description: Black solid

(b) Melting-point: Above 180°C (decomposition)

(c) Solubility: Soluble in water (120 mg/l at room temperature), acetone, chloroform, pyridine and acetonitrile

1.4 Technical products and impurities

Ferbam is available in the US as dusts containing 0.6-25% of the chemical, as wettable powders containing 3-98% and as a flowable formulation containing 42%. In Japan, ferbam is available as a technical product containing at least 95% of the chemical (Japanese Ministry of Agriculture & Forestry, 1975).

2.   Production, Use, Occurrence and Analysis

For important background information on this section, see preamble, p. 15.

2.1 Production and use

Ferbam was first prepared and evaluated as a fungicide in about 1931 (Tisdale & Williams, 1934). It can be prepared by the reaction of dimethyl-amine with carbon disulphide in the presence of sodium hydroxide followed by addition of a ferric salt, such as ferric chloride (Kent, 1974). This is believed to be the method used in the commercial production of ferbam.

Ferbam has been produced commercially in the US since 1945 (US Tariff Commission, 1947). US production reached a maximum level of 1.4 million kg in 1961 (US Tariff Commission, 1962); in 1968, the last year for which production quantities were reported, 0.8 million kg ferbam were produced (US Department of Agriculture, 1972); in recent years, only 1 or 2 companies have produced it. Total US exports of all dithiocarbamate formulations were 6.7 million kg in 1974 (US Department of Commerce, 1975).

Ferbam is produced by one company in The Netherlands (Berg, 1975); one producer in France and one in the UK have an estimated total annual production of less than 1 million kg.

One company in Japan began producing ferbam in 1970. The quantity produced has decreased from 28.6 thousand kg in 1970 to only 700 kg in 1974 (Japanese Ministry of Agriculture & Forestry, 1975).

In the US, ferbam is used as a fungicide to control diseases of plants, particularly those affecting apples and tobacco (Berg, 1975), and is registered for use on about 75 agricultural and ornamental plants (US Environ-

122

mental Protection Agency, 1973). In 1971, 356 thousand kg were used on agricultural crops in the US (US Department of Agriculture, 1974).

In Europe, ferbam is utilized as follows: fungicide (80%), rubber accelerator (19%) and plastics pro-degradant (1%). In Japan, it is used on apples and citrus fruits (Japanese Ministry of Agriculture & Forestry, 1975).

A residue tolerance of 7 mg/kg has been established in the US for about 60 raw agricultural commodities (US Code of Federal Regulations, 1974), and many US commodities may bear residues of ferbam approaching this level. According to the US Occupational Safety and Health Administration health standards for air contaminants, an employee's exposure to ferbam should not exceed 15 mg/m³ in the workplace air during any eight-hour workshift for a forty-hour week (US Code of Federal Regulations, 1975).

In December 1974, the Joint Meeting of the FAO Working Party of Experts on Pesticide Residues and the WHO Expert Committee on Pesticide Residues established a revised temporary acceptable daily intake for man of 0-0.005 mg/kg bw for all dithiocarbamate fungicides (WHO, 1975a,b).

2.2 Occurrence

Ferbam is not known to occur as a natural product. For information on the levels of ethylenethiourea, a possible breakdown product, that may be found on raw agricultural products, see IARC (1974).

As part of the 'Total Diet Program' of the US Food and Drug Administration, 360 composite food samples were collected annually during the period 1964-1970, prepared as for consumption and analysed for dithiocarbamate content. A maximum of 4 composites contained detectable levels of dithiocarbamates in any single year (Corneliussen, 1972), and in at least one year no dithiocarbamate was detected. On the basis of these results, analysis for dithiocarbamates in this programme was discontinued after 1970 (Manske & Corneliussen, 1974).

2.3 Analysis

Methods for the chromatographic analysis of carbamates, including dithiocarbamate pesticides, have been reviewed (Fishbein & Zielinski, 1967).

Ferbam residues have been determined by polarography, with a sensitivity of 80 µg/ml (Supin *et al.*, 1973) or of 10^{-7} M (Budnikov *et al.*, 1974). The voltametric behaviour of ferbam has also been studied (Golding *et al.*, 1974) and might provide the basis for an analytical method. A rapid colorimetric method for the estimation of ferbam residues on grains allows recoveries of 91-100% at levels of 10-1000 µg (Rangaswamy *et al.*, 1970).

3. Biological Data Relevant to the Evaluation of Carcinogenic Risk to Man

3.1 Carcinogenicity and related studies in animals

(a) Oral administration

Mouse: Groups of 18 male and 18 female (C57BL/6xC3H/Anf)F_1 mice and 18 male and 18 female (C57BL/6xAKR)F_1 mice received commercial ferbam (97% pure) according to the following schedule: 10 mg/kg bw in gelatine at 7 days of age by stomach tube and the same amount (not adjusted for increasing body weight) daily up to 4 weeks of age; subsequently, the mice were given 32 mg ferbam per kg of diet. The dose given was the maximum tolerated dose for infant and young mice but not necessarily so for adults. The experiment was terminated when the animals were about 78 weeks of age, at which time 16, 16, 16 and 15 mice in the four groups, respectively, were still alive. Tumour incidences were compared with those observed among 79-90 necropsied mice of each sex and strain, which either had been untreated or had received gelatine only: the incidences were not significantly greater (P>0.05) for any tumour type in any sex-strain subgroup or in the combined sexes of either strain (Innes *et al.*, 1969; NTIS, 1968).

Rat: Four groups of 25 4-week old rats of each sex were fed 0, 25, 250 or 2500 mg ferbam per kg of diet for 2 years. Controls lived for 600-700 days; median length of survival among rats given either 25 or 250 mg ferbam per kg of diet was not altered, whereas at the highest dose lifespan was about 430 days. There were 12 tumours in treated animals, and 7 in control rats; these were reported to be unrelated to dose. Tumour sites were not indicated (Hodge *et al.*, 1956).

(b) Subcutaneous administration

Mouse: Groups of 18 male and 18 female (C57BL/6xC3H/Anf)F_1 mice and 18 male and 18 female (C57BL/6xAKR)F_1 mice were given single s.c. injections of 100 mg/kg bw commercial ferbam (95% pure) in 0.5% gelatine at 28 days of age and were observed until they were about 78 weeks of age, at which time 15, 17, 18 and 16 mice in the four groups, respectively, were still alive. Tumour incidences were compared with those in groups of 141, 154, 161 and 157 untreated or vehicle-injected controls that were necropsied. Incidences were not increased (P>0.05) for any tumour type in any sex-strain subgroup or in the combined sexes of either strain (NTIS, 1968) [The Working Group noted that a negative result obtained with a single subcutaneous injection may not be an adequate basis for discounting carcinogenicity].

3.2 Other relevant biological data

(a) Experimental systems

In short- and long-term feeding studies in rats given diets containing 25-2500 mg/kg ferbam, apart from non-neoplastic brain changes in rats given the highest dose, no adverse effects were seen (Hodge et al., 1952, 1956).

Approximately 40-70% of an oral dose of ferbam was absorbed from the gastrointestinal tract of rats during a 24-hour period. In rats that received ^{35}S-ferbam, 18% of the ^{35}S was excreted in the exhaled air as carbon disulphide and 23% in the urine. In those given [dimethyl-^{14}C]-ferbam, 43% of the radioactivity was found in the urine as dimethylamine and dimethyldithiocarbamate glucuronide (Hodgson et al., 1975).

The combination of ferbam with ethanol caused accumulation of acetaldehyde in the blood (van Logten, 1972). Ferbam reacts with nitrite to form N-nitrosodimethylamine (Sen et al., 1974).

When pregnant rats were dosed with [dimethyl-^{14}C]-ferbam, a small amount of radioactivity crossed the placenta and accumulated in the foetuses. Radioactivity was also secreted into the milk of lactating rats given [dimethyl-^{14}C]-ferbam and was in turn excreted in the urine of the pups (Hodgson et al., 1974, 1975).

Administration of 150 mg/kg bw/day ferbam to pregnant rats on days 6-15 of gestation caused some foetal deaths, increased resorption, decreased foetal weight and produced a slight increase in the number of animals with soft and skeletal tissue abnormalities (Minor *et al.*, 1974).

Prasad & Pramer (1968) reported colour mutants and reverse mutations in *Aspergillus niger*; metabolic activation systems were not used in these tests.

(b) Man

No data were available to the Working Group, but for a discussion of the interaction of compounds such as ferbam with ethanol in the blood, see 'General Remarks on Carbamates, Thiocarbamates and Carbazides', pp. 28-29.

3.3 Case reports and epidemiological studies

No data were available to the Working Group.

4. Comments on Data Reported and Evaluation

4.1 Animal data

Ferbam has been tested by oral administration in mice and rats and by single subcutaneous injection in mice. Although no carcinogenic effect was observed in these tests, the available data are insufficient for an evaluation of the carcinogenicity of this compound to be made.

Ferbam can react with nitrite under mildly acid conditions, simulating those in the human stomach, to form N-nitrosodimethylamine, which has been shown to be carcinogenic in seven animal species (IARC, 1972).

4.2 Human data

No case reports or epidemiological studies were available to the Working Group.

5. References

Berg, G.L., ed. (1975) Farm Chemicals Handbook 1975, Willoughby, Ohio, Meister, p. D93

Budnikov, G.K., Toropova, V.F., Ulakhovich, N.A. & Viter, I.P. (1974) Electrochemical behavior of dithiocarbamates on a mercury electrode. III. Polarographic study of fungicides of dithiocarbamate type in organic solvents. Zh. analyt. Khim., 29, 1204-1209

Corneliussen, P.E. (1972) Pesticide residues in total diet samples. Pest. Monit. J., 5, 313-330

Fishbein, L. & Zielinski, W.L., Jr (1967) Chromatography of carbamates. Chromat. Rev., 9, 37-101

Golding, R.M., Lehtonen, K. & Ralph, B.J. (1974) Voltammetry of tris(N,N-diorganodithiocarbamato) iron (III) complexes in acetone. J. inorg. nucl. Chem., 36, 2047-2050

Hodge, H.C., Maynard, E.A., Downs, W., Blanchet, H.J., Jr & Jones, C.K. (1952) Acute and short-term oral toxicity tests of ferric dimethyldithiocarbamate (Ferbam) and zinc dimethyldithiocarbamate (Ziram). J. Amer. pharm. Ass., 41, 662-665

Hodge, H.C., Maynard, E.A., Downs, W.L., Coye, R.D., Jr & Steadman, L.T. (1956) Chronic oral toxicity of ferric dimethyldithiocarbamate (Ferbam) and zinc dimethyldithiocarbamate (Ziram). J. Pharmacol. exp. Ther., 118, 174-181

Hodgson, J.R., Castles, T.R., Murrill, E. & Lee, C.-C. (1974) Distribution, excretion and metabolism of the fungicide ferbam in rats. Fed. Proc., 33, 537

Hodgson, J.R., Hoch, J.C., Castles, T.R., Helton, D.O. & Lee, C.-C. (1975) Metabolism and disposition of ferbam in the rat. Toxicol. appl. Pharmacol., 33, 505-513

IARC (1972) IARC Monographs on the Evaluation of Carcinogenic Risk of Chemicals to Man, 1, Lyon, pp. 95-106

IARC (1974) IARC Monographs on the Evaluation of Carcinogenic Risk of Chemicals to Man, 7, Some Anti-thyroid and Related Substances, Nitrofurans and Industrial Chemicals, Lyon, pp. 45-52

Innes, J.R.M., Ulland, B.M., Valerio, M.G., Petrucelli, L., Fishbein, L., Hart, E.R., Pallotta, A.J., Bates, R.R., Falk, H.L., Gart, J.J., Klein, M., Mitchell, I. & Peters, J. (1969) Bioassay of pesticides and industrial chemicals for tumorigenicity in mice: a preliminary note. J. nat. Cancer Inst., 42, 1101-1114

Japanese Ministry of Agriculture and Forestry (1975) Noyaku Yoran (Agri-
    cultural Chemicals Annual), 1975, Division of Plant Disease Prevention,
    Tokyo, Takeo Endo, pp. 17, 18, 20, 267, 268, 275

Kent, J.A., ed. (1974) Riegel's Handbook of Industrial Chemistry, 7th ed.,
    New York, Van Nostrand-Reinhold, pp. 634-635

van Logten, M.J. (1972) De Dithiocarbamaat-Alcohol-Reactie bij de Rat,
    Terborg, The Netherlands, Bedrijf FA. Lammers, p. 40

Manske, D.D. & Corneliussen, P.E. (1974) Pesticide residues in total diet
    samples. VII. Pest. Monit. J., 8, 110-114

Minor, J.L., Russell, J.Q. & Lee, C.-C. (1974) Reproduction and teratology
    studies with the fungicide ferbam. Toxicol. appl. Pharmacol., 29, 120

NTIS (National Technical Information Service) (1968) Evaluation of Carcino-
    genic, Teratogenic and Mutagenic Activities of Selected Pesticides and
    Industrial Chemicals, Vol. 1, Carcinogenic Study, Washington DC, US
    Department of Commerce

Prasad, I. & Pramer, D. (1968) Genetic effects of ferbam on *Aspergillus
    niger* and *Allium cepa*. Phytopathology, 58, 1188-1189

Rangaswamy, J.R., Poornima, P. & Majumder, S.K. (1970) Rapid colorimetric
    method for estimation of ferbam and ziram residues on grains. J. Ass.
    off. analyt. Chem., 53, 1043-1044

Sen, N.P., Donaldson, B.A. & Charbonneau, C. (1974) Formation of nitroso-
    dimethylamine from the interaction of certain pesticides and nitrite.
    In: Bogovski, P. & Walker, E.A., eds, *N*-Nitroso Compounds in the
    Environment, Lyon, IARC (IARC Scientific Publications No. 9), pp. 75-79

Stecher, P.G., ed. (1968) The Merck Index, 8th ed., Rahway, NJ, Merck &
    Co., p. 451

Supin, G.S., Klisenko, M.A. & Vekshtein, M.S. (1973) Polarographic deter-
    mination of residual amounts of fungicide as dithiocarbonic acid
    derivatives. Khim. Sel. Khoz., 11, 840-842

Tisdale, W.H. & Williams, I. (1934) Disinfectant. US Patent 1,972,961,
    September 11, to E.I. du Pont de Nemours and Co.

US Code of Federal Regulations (1974) Protection of Environment, Title 40,
    part. 180.114, Washington DC, US Government Printing Office, pp. 248-249

US Code of Federal Regulations (1975) Air Contaminants, Title 29,
    part. 1910.1000, Washington DC, US Government Printing Office, p. 61

US Department of Agriculture (1972) The Pesticide Review 1971, Washington DC,
    US Government Printing Office, p. 18

US Department of Agriculture (1974) Farmers' Use of Pesticides in 1971, Quantities, Economic Research Service, Agricultural Economic Report, No. 252, Washington DC, US Government Printing Office, p. 25

US Department of Commerce (1975) US Exports, FT 4101, December 1974, Bureau of the Census, Washington DC, US Government Printing Office, pp. 2-135-2-136

US Environmental Protection Agency (1973) EPA Compendium of Registered Pesticides, Vol. II, Fungicides and Nematicides, Washington DC, US Government Printing Office, part. I, pp. F-01-00.01-F-01-00.10

US Tariff Commission (1947) Synthetic Organic Chemicals, US Production and Sales, 1945, Report No. 157, Second Series, Washington DC, US Government Printing Office, p. 186

US Tariff Commission (1962) Synthetic Organic Chemicals, US Production and Sales, 1961, TC Publication 72, Washington DC, US Government Printing Office, p. 166

WHO (1975a) 1974 Evaluations of some pesticide residues in food. Wld Hlth Org. Pest. Res. Ser., No. 4, pp. 261-263

WHO (1975b) Pesticide residues in food. Report of the 1974 Joint Meeting of the FAO Working Party of Experts on Pesticide Residues and the WHO Expert Committee on Pesticide Residues. Wld Hlth Org. techn. Rep. Ser., No. 574, pp. 26-28

LEDATE

1. Chemical and Physical Data

1.1 Synonyms and trade names

Chem. Abstr. Reg. Serial No.: 19010-66-3

Chem. Abstr. Name: Bis(dimethylcarbamodithioato-S,S')lead

Lead dimethyldithiocarbamate

1.2 Chemical formula and molecular weight

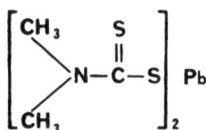

$$\left[\begin{array}{c} CH_3 \\ \diagdown N-C-S \\ CH_3 \end{array} \begin{array}{c} S \\ \| \\ \end{array} \right]_2 Pb$$

$C_6H_{12}N_2PbS_4$ Mol. wt: 447.6

1.3 Chemical and physical properties of the pure substance

No data were available to the Working Group.

1.4 Technical products and impurities

Ledate powder is available commercially in the US with the following specifications: white powder; density, 2.43 ± 0.03; particle size, 99.9% passes through a 100-mesh screen; lead content, 45.5-47.5%; melting-point, above 310°C; moisture (at 100-105°C), 1% max. (Anon., 1975a).

For rubber processing, ledate is available commercially in the US in the form of rods with similar specifications (Anon., 1975b). It is also available as a paste with 30% light oil and as a dispersion with 25% polyisobutylene binder (Anon., 1975a).

2. Production, Use, Occurrence and Analysis

For important background information on this section, see preamble, p. 15.

2.1 Production and use

Ledate can be prepared from lead acetate and potassium dimethyl-dithiocarbamate (IARC, 1972; Jensen *et al.*, 1971). Commercial production in the US was first reported in 1934 (US Tariff Commission, 1936); in 1974, only one manufacturer reported production (US International Trade Commission, 1975). It is estimated that less than 1 million kg are produced annually in the Benelux countries, Italy and the UK.

Ledate is used in the rubber-processing industry as an accelerator for high-speed, high-temperature vulcanization. It is used in compounding natural, styrene-butadiene, isobutylene-isoprene, isoprene and butadiene rubbers. It is effective under continuous curing conditions and is generally used with thiazole modifiers (Anon., 1975a).

2.2 Occurrence

Ledate is not known to occur as a natural product.

2.3 Analysis

Methods for the chromatographic analysis of carbamates, including thiocarbamates, have been reviewed (Fishbein & Zielinski, 1967) A thin-layer chromatographic-spectrophotofluorimetric method (van Hoof & Heyndrickx, 1973) is suitable for the analysis of a variety of metal dithiocarbamates, although it was not applied to ledate itself.

An investigation of the electrochemical behaviour of metal dithio-carbamates, including ledate, has been reported (Budnikov *et al.*, 1974).

3. Biological Data Relevant to the Evaluation
of Carcinogenic Risk to Man

3.1 Carcinogenicity and related studies in animals

(a) Oral administration

Mouse: Groups of 18 male and 18 female (C57BL/6xC3H/Anf)F_1 mice and
18 male and 18 female (C57BL/6xAKR)F_1 mice received commercial ledate
(m.p. >310°C) according to the following schedule: 46.4 mg/kg bw in
gelatine at 7 days of age by stomach tube and the same amount (not adjusted
for increasing body weight) daily up to 4 weeks of age; subsequently,
the mice were given 130 mg ledate per kg of diet. The dose was the
maximum tolerated dose for infant and young mice but not necessarily so
for adults. The experiment was terminated when the animals were about
78 weeks of age, at which time 16, 16, 17 and 18 mice in the four groups,
respectively, were still alive. Tumour incidences were compared with
those in 79-90 necropsied mice of each sex and strain, which had been
untreated or had received gelatine only. Tumours developed in 7/16
necropsied males (1 malignant lymphoma, 1 hepatoma, 5 reticulum-cell
sarcomas) and 1/18 necropsied females (1 bone tumour) of the first strain
and in 2/17 males (2 pulmonary adenomas) of the second strain. The
incidence of reticulum-cell sarcomas in males of the first strain was
significantly different from that in controls (5/16 *versus* 5/79) [P<0.01]
(Innes *et al.*, 1969; NTIS, 1968).

(b) Subcutaneous administration

Mouse: Groups of 18 male and 18 female (C57BL/6xC3H/Anf)F_1 mice and
18 male and 18 female (C57BL/6xAKR)F_1 mice were given single s.c. injections
of 1000 mg/kg bw commercial ledate (m.p. >310°C) in 0.5% gelatine on the
28th day of life and were observed until they were about 78 weeks of age,
at which time 15, 18, 18 and 15 mice in the four groups, respectively,
were still alive. Tumour incidences were compared with those in groups
of 141, 154, 161 and 157 untreated or vehicle-injected controls that were
necropsied. Incidences were not increased (P>0.05) for any tumour type
in any sex-strain subgroup or in the combined sexes of either strain
(NTIS, 1968) [The Working Group noted that a negative result obtained

with a single s.c. injection may not be an adequate basis for discounting carcinogenicity].

3.2 Other relevant biological data

No data were available to the Working Group.

3.3 Case reports and epidemiological studies

No data were available to the Working Group.

4. Comments on Data Reported and Evaluation

4.1 Animal data

Ledate has been tested by oral administration and by single subcutaneous injection in two strains of mice. Although an increase in the incidence of reticulum-cell sarcomas was observed in males of one strain following oral administration of the compound, the available data are insufficient for evaluation of its carcinogenicity.

4.2 Human data

No case reports or epidemiological studies were available to the Working Group.

5. References

Anon. (1975a) Materials and Compounding Ingredients for Rubber, New York, Bill Communications, pp. 42, 49, 51

Anon. (1975b) Ledate®, Color Rodform®, Norwalk, Connecticut, R.T. Vanderbilt Co.

Budnikov, G.K., Ulakhovich, N.A., Viter, I.P. & Kolesnikova, L.V. (1974) Effect of the adsorption of a depolarizer on the polarographic reduction of metal dithiocarbamates in organic solvents. J. gen. Chem. (USSR), 44, 730-737

Fishbein, L. & Zielinski, W.L., Jr (1967) Chromatography of carbamates. Chromat. Rev., 9, 37-101

van Hoof, F. & Heyndrickx, A. (1973) Thin layer chromatographic-spectro-photofluorimetric methods for the determination of dithio- and thiol-carbamates after hydrolysis and coupling with NBD-Cl. Ghent. Rijks-univ. Fac. Landbl. Med., 38, 911-916

IARC (1972) IARC Monographs on the Evaluation of Carcinogenic Risk of Chemicals to Man, 9, Some Aziridines, N-, S- and O-Mustards and Selenium, Lyon, pp. 40-50

Innes, J.R.M., Ulland, B.M., Valerio, M.G., Petrucelli, L., Fishbein, L., Hart, E.R., Pallotta, A.J., Bates, R.R., Falk, H.L., Gart, J.J., Klein, M., Mitchell, I. & Peters, J. (1969) Bioassay of pesticides and industrial chemicals for tumorigenicity in mice: a preliminary note. J. nat. Cancer Inst., 42, 1101-1114

Jensen, K.A., Dahl, B.M., Nielsen, P.H. & Borch, G. (1971) Tentative assignment of fundamental vibrations of thio- and selenocarboxylates. II. The dimethyldithiocarbamate ion. Acta chem. scand., 25, 2029-2038

NTIS (National Technical Information Service) (1968) Evaluation of Carcino-genic, Teratogenic and Mutagenic Activities of Selected Pesticides and Industrial Chemicals, Vol. 1, Carcinogenic Study, Washington DC, US Department of Commerce

US International Trade Commission (1975) Synthetic Organic Chemicals, US Production and Sales of Rubber-Processing Chemicals, 1974 Preliminary, Washington DC, US Government Printing Office, p. 8

US Tariff Commission (1936) Dyes and Other Synthetic Organic Chemicals in the US, 1934, Report No. 101, Second Series, Washington DC, US Government Printing Office, p. 66

MANEB

1. Chemical and Physical Data

1.1 Synonyms and trade names

Chem. Abstr. Reg. Serial No.: 12427-38-2

Chem. Abstr. Name: {[1,2-Ethanediylbis(carbamodithioato)] (2-)}-manganese

1,2-Ethanediylbiscarbamodithioic acid, manganese complex; 1,2-ethanediylbiscarbamodithioic acid, manganese (2+) salt (1:1); 1,2-ethanediylbismaneb, manganese(2+)salt(1:1); ethylenebis(dithio-carbamato), manganese; ethylenebis(dithiocarbamic acid), manganese salt; 1,2-ethylenediylbis(carbamodithioato)manganese; manebe; manganese ethylene bisdithiocarbamate

Chloroble M; Dithane M22; Dithane M-22 Special; Kypman 80; Maneb 80; Maneba; Manebgan; Manesan; Manzate; Manzate D; Polyram M; Rhodianebe; Sopranebe; Sup'R Flo; Trimangol; Vancide Maneb 80

1.2 Chemical formula and molecular weight

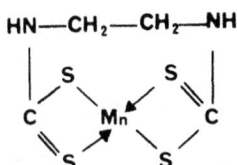

$C_4H_6MnN_2S_4$ Mol. wt: 265.3

1.3 Chemical and physical properties of the substance

From Stecher (1968), unless otherwise specified

(a) Description: Crystals from ethanol

(b) Melting-point: Decomposes before melting (Association of American Pesticide Control Officials, Inc., 1962)

(c) Solubility: Moderately soluble in water; soluble in chloroform and pyridine

1.4 Technical products and impurities

Maneb is available in the US as a wettable powder, containing 80% of the chemical, and in formulations, which also contain a small amount of an inorganic zinc salt (Berg, 1975).

Many commercial ethylenebisdithiocarbamate samples, including maneb, contain ethylenethiourea (ETU) (Bontoyan *et al.*, 1972). Bontoyan & Looker (1973) studied the initial ETU contents of various ethylenebisdithiocar-bamate products and the levels after storage at 88°C. The initial ETU content in specific formulations of 'maneb, 80%' varied between 0.05 and 1.26%; after 39 days of storage ETU levels varied between 0.58 and 14.54%.

2. Production, Use, Occurrence and Analysis

For important background information on this section, see preamble, p. 15. A review on maneb has been published by the US Environmental Protection Agency (1974).

2.1 Production and use

Maneb can be prepared by the reaction of ethylenediamine with carbon disulphide in the presence of sodium hydroxide to produce the sodium salt, which is then treated with a manganese salt (e.g., manganese sulphate) to precipitate maneb (US Environmental Protection Agency, 1974).

Maneb was introduced as an agricultural fungicide in the US in 1950. Two US companies produced an estimated 5.5 million kg of maneb in 1972, and exports were estimated to be 2 million kg (US Environmental Protection Agency, 1974). It is also produced in Israel and in The Netherlands (Berg, 1975); 1.5 million kg are estimated to be produced annually in both France and Italy, and less than 1 million kg each in the Federal Republic of Germany, Spain and the UK.

In Japan, production of maneb was started in 1964; two companies now produce it, and in 1974 production reached a level of 1.9 million kg.

Imports from France, Israel, The Netherlands and the US amounted to about 800 thousand kg in 1974, down from about 900 thousand kg in 1973. There have been no exports from Japan since 1972 when minor quantities were exported to India, Korea, The People's Republic of China, Taiwan and Thailand (Japanese Ministry of Agriculture & Forestry, 1975).

Maneb is used exclusively as a broad spectrum contact fungicide and is registered for use on over 46 crops in the US. The principal diseases controlled by maneb are early and late blight of potato and tomato, downy mildew and anthracnose on a number of vegetables and the so-called 'rot' diseases of fruits such as apricots, peaches and grapes. It is also used for seed treatment of small grains, such as wheat (US Environmental Protection Agency, 1974).

In 1971, 1.7 million kg were used on US agricultural crops (US Department of Agriculture, 1974); in 1974, of about 70 thousand kg used in California, one third was on head lettuce (California Department of Food & Agriculture, 1975). In Italy, an estimated 2 million kg are utilized annually. In Japan, over half of the 2.1 million kg maneb used in 1974 was used on paddy-field rice, about one-third was used on citrus fruits, and the remainder was used on melons and vegetables (Japanese Ministry of Agriculture & Forestry, 1975).

Residue tolerances on raw agricultural products in the US are generally in the range of 2-10 mg/kg, with the exceptions of 0.1, 15 and 45 mg/kg for almonds and potatoes, bananas and sugar-beet tops, respectively (US Code of Federal Regulations, 1974).

In December 1974, the Joint Meeting of the FAO Working Party of Experts on Pesticide Residues and the WHO Expert Committee on Pesticide Residues established a revised temporary acceptable daily intake for man of 0-0.005 mg/kg bw for all dithiocarbamate fungicides (WHO, 1975a,b).

2.2 Occurrence

Maneb is not known to occur as a natural product.

As part of the 'Total Diet Program' of the US Food and Drug Administration, 360 composite food samples were collected annually during the period 1964-1970, prepared as for consumption and analysed for dithiocarbamate content. A maximum of 4 composites contained detectable levels of dithiocarbamates in any single year (Corneliussen, 1972), and in at least one year, no dithiocarbamate was detected. On the basis of these results, analysis for dithiocarbamates in this programme was discontinued after 1970 (Manske & Corneliussen, 1974).

The significance of maneb as a residue on agricultural products is enhanced by reports that the cooking of foods containing ethylenebisdithiocarbamate residues would result in degradation to form ETU; thus, cooking of vegetables containing residues of maneb near the tolerance level would result in the formation of ETU (Blazquez, 1973; Watts *et al.*, 1974). For information on the levels of ETU which can be found on raw agricultural products, see IARC (1974).

2.3 Analysis

Three reviews which include methods for the analysis of maneb have been published (Fishbein, 1975; Fishbein & Zielinski, 1967; Zweig & Sherma, 1972).

Maneb has been determined following its hydrolysis with hydrochloric acid containing stannous chloride; the resulting ethylenediamine is recovered on an ion-exchange column and determined by gas chromatography as the bis-trifluoroacetate. The limit of detection was 0.1 mg/kg (Newsome, 1974). A screening procedure has been developed for dithiocarbamate residues in food involving head-space analysis of the carbon disulphide produced on hydrolysis. The carbon disulphide was determined by gas chromatography, using a flame photometric detector. Recoveries of maneb added to samples at the 7 mg/kg level were 70-95% (McLeod & McCully, 1969). Carbon disulphide formation with a colorimetric end determination (Keppel, 1969) was used by Yip *et al.* (1971) to determine maneb residues in field-sprayed lettuce and kale and by Howard & Yip (1971) to study the stability of maneb, zineb and Dithane M-22 added to kale. Polarographic methods have also been used: Budnikov *et al.* (1974) showed that 10^{-7} M levels of manganese compounds can be determined.

Stevenson (1972) has described a test based on the colour developed by acid dithizone, which depends on the type and concentration of metal present. However, the presence of a dithiocarbamate must be established separately, using conventional procedures.

3. Biological Data Relevant to the Evaluation of Carcinogenic Risk to Man

3.1 Carcinogenicity and related studies in animals

(a) Oral administration

Mouse: Groups of 18 male and 18 female (C57BL/6xC3H/Anf)F$_1$ mice and 18 male and 18 female (C57BL/6xAKR)F$_1$ mice received commercial maneb (96% pure) according to the following schedule: 46.4 mg/kg bw in gelatine at 7 days of age by stomach tube and the same amount (not adjusted for increasing body weight) daily up to 4 weeks of age; subsequently, the mice were given 158 mg maneb per kg of diet. The dose was the maximum tolerated dose for infant and young mice but not necessarily so for adults. The experiment was terminated when the animals were about 78 weeks of age, at which time 16, 15, 18 and 18 mice in the four groups, respectively, were still alive. Tumour incidences were compared with those observed among 79-90 necropsied mice of each sex and strain, which either had been untreated or had received gelatine only: the incidences were not significantly greater (P>0.05) for any type of tumour in any sex-strain subgroup or in the combined sexes of either strain (Innes et al., 1969; NTIS, 1968).

A group of 200 C57BL mice was given 6 weekly administrations of maneb by stomach tube, each dose corresponding to 500 mg/kg bw. The mice were killed at intervals of up to 9 months; of 42 survivors killed at 9 months, 4 had lung adenomas. The incidence in untreated controls was 0/44 (P>0.05). Among similarly treated strain A mice, 23/42 had lung adenomas after 9 months, compared with 12/45 controls [P<0.01] (Balin, 1970).

Rat: Of 60 random-bred rats given twice weekly doses of 335 mg/kg bw maneb (82.6% pure) in water by stomach tube for lifespan, 6 were still alive after 22 months; 1 rat developed a subcutaneous rhabdomyosarcoma and another a mammary carcinoma. One fibrosarcoma was observed among 46 untreated control rats still alive after 22 months (Andrianova & Alekseev, 1970).

141

(b) Subcutaneous administration

Mouse: Groups of 18 male and 18 female (C57BL/6xC3H/Anf)F$_1$ mice and
18 male and 18 female (C57BL/6xAKR)F$_1$ mice were given single s.c. injections
of 100 mg/kg bw commercial maneb (96% pure) in 0.5% gelatine on the 28th
day of life and were observed until they were about 78 weeks of age, at
which time 17, 18, 18 and 17 mice in the four groups, respectively, were
still alive. Tumour incidences were compared with those of groups of 141,
154, 161 and 157 untreated or vehicle-injected controls that were necropsied.
Incidences were not increased (P>0.05) for any tumour type in any sex-strain
subgroup or in the combined sexes of either strain (NTIS, 1968) [The Working
Group noted that a negative result obtained with a single s.c. injection may
not be an adequate basis for discounting carcinogenicity].

Rat: Of 48 random-bred rats given single s.c. injections of 12.5 mg/kg
bw maneb (82.6% pure) in paraffin, 4 were still alive after 22 months, and
3 developed malignant tumours (2 fibrosarcomas and 1 thyroid carcinoma).
One fibrosarcoma was seen in 46 control rats which did not receive paraffin
pellets and were still alive at 22 months (Andrianova & Alekseev, 1970).

3.2 Other relevant biological data

(a) Experimental systems

The oral LD$_{50}$ of maneb in mice is 4.1 g/kg bw; that in rats has been
reported as 4.5 g/kg bw (Engst et al., 1971) and 6.7 g/kg bw (Berg, 1975).
Maneb intoxication increased thyroid function in rats (Ivanova et al.,
1967; Ivanova-Chemishanska et al., 1971).

In rats, 55% of an oral dose of ^{14}C-maneb was excreted in the urine
and faeces (36% in the urine) within 3 days. After 24 hours, the body
organs contained 1.2% of the dose as maneb metabolites, and on day 5, less
than 0.18%; ethylenediamine, ethylenebisthiuram monosulphide and ETU
were present in the urine and faeces (Seidler et al., 1970) [The authors
do not appear to have measured pulmonary excretion, which is likely to
account for much of the remainder of the dose].

Maneb (1) (Scheme 1) is hydrolysed by acids into ethylenediamine (2)
and carbon disulphide, and this reaction may take place under the acid

142

SCHEME 1

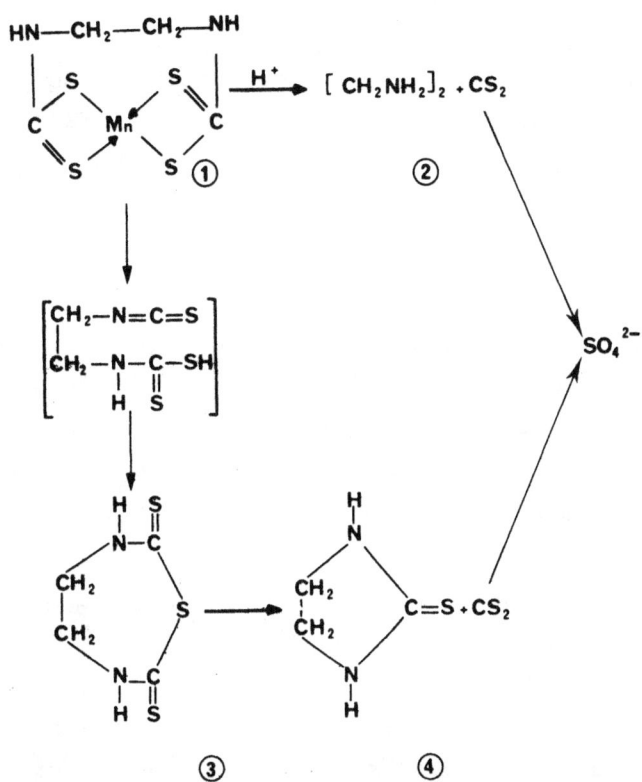

conditions of the stomach, accounting for some of the carbon disulphide that is excreted in exhaled air; the remainder arises from the transformation of ethylene bisthiuram monosulphide (3) into ETU (4). Some of the absorbed (2) would be oxidized to glycine and oxalic acid and, ultimately, to carbon dioxide. The rest of the ethylenediamine (2) is excreted in the urine, together with (4) and inorganic sulphate, but ethylene bisthiuram monosulphide (3) is excreted in the faeces (Seidler *et al.*, 1970).

Groups of 10 male and 10 female rats were given 1.4 g/kg bw or 700 mg/kg bw maneb twice weekly for $4\frac{1}{2}$ months. There was a moderately high incidence of stillbirths and of imperfect skull development, but the actual numbers compared with those among controls is not stated (Kaloyanova *et al.*, 1967).

Female rats were given 50 mg/kg bw as a suspension in milk on every other day during pregnancy; increased numbers of embryonic deaths, resorptions, stillborn young and neonates incapable of survival were observed. The unfavourable effect of maneb on the course of gestation was apparent in 21% of pregnancies, compared with a 12% background of untoward events among the control animals. In addition, immature female and male rats (80-100 g bw) were administered 50 mg/kg bw/day for 1 month. After $2\frac{1}{2}$ months, control males were mated with exposed females and *vice versa*. A decline in fertility was observed in both sexes, but this effect was reversible within $3\frac{1}{2}$ months (Marcon, 1969).

When single oral doses of 1, 2 or 4 g/kg bw were administered to pregnant rats on day 11 or 13 of pregnancy, congenital abnormalities were induced in 12-100% of the foetuses; no congenital abnormalities were observed with 0.5 mg/kg bw (Petrova-Vergieva & Ivanova-Chemishanska, 1973). Similar tests with maneb have been made by Shtenberg *et al.* (1969) and by Antonovich *et al.* (1972).

A slight increase in the number of chromosomal aberrations in metaphases of bone-marrow cells was observed in mice treated with 100 mg/kg bw orally (Antonovich *et al.*, 1971).

(b) Man

No data were available to the Working Group.

144

(c) Carcinogenicity of metabolites

ETU (4) (Scheme 1) produced thyroid carcinomas in rats and increased the incidence of liver-cell tumours in two strains of mice after its oral administration (IARC, 1974).

3.3 Case reports and epidemiological studies

No data were available to the Working Group.

4. Comments on Data Reported and Evaluation

4.1 Animal data

Maneb has been tested in mice and rats by oral administration and by single subcutaneous injection. Its oral administration produced an increased incidence of lung tumours in mice of one strain, but no increase was observed in three other strains. The studies in rats cannot be evaluated due to the small numbers of surviving animals. No evaluation of the carcinogenicity of this compound can be made.

4.2 Human data

No case reports or epidemiological studies were available to the Working Group.

5. References

Andrianova, M.M. & Alekseev, I.V. (1970) On the carcinogenic properties of the pesticides sevine, maneb, ciram and cineb. Vop. Pitan., 29, 71-74

Antonovich, E.A. Chepynoga, O.P., Chernov, O.V., Rjazanova, P.A., Vekshtein, M.S., Martson, V.S., Martson, L.V., Samosh, L.V., Pilinskaya, M.A., Kurinny, L.I., Balin, P.N., Khitsenko, I.I., Zastavnjuk, N.P. & Zaolorozhnaja, N.A. (1971) Toxicity of dithiocarbamates and their fate in warmblooded animals. In: Antonovich, E.A., Bojanovska, A., Engst, P. et al., eds, Proceedings of the Symposium on Toxicology and Analytical Chemistry of Dithiocarbamates, Dubrovnic, 1970, Beograd, pp. 3-20

Antonovich, E.A., Chernov, O.V., Samosh, L.V., Martson, L.V., Pilinskaya, M.A., Kurinny, L.I., Vekshtein, M.S., Martson, V.S., Balin, P.N. & Khitsenko, I.I. (1972) A comparative toxicological assessment of dithiocarbamates. Gig. i Sanit., 50, 25-30

Association of American Pesticide Control Officials, Inc. (1962) Pesticide Chemicals Official Compendium, Box HH, University P.O., College Park, Maryland, p. 193

Balin, P.N. (1970) Experimental data on the blastomogenic activity of the fungicide maneb. Vrach. Delo, 4, 21-24

Berg, G.L., ed. (1975) Farm Chemicals Handbook 1975, Willoughby, Ohio, Meister, p. D 124

Blazquez, C.H. (1973) Residue determination of ethylenethiourea (2-imidazolidinethione) from tomato foliage, soil and water. J. agric. Fd Chem., 21, 330-332

Bontoyan, W.R. & Looker, J.B. (1973) Degradation of commercial ethylene bisdithiocarbamate formulations to ethylenethiourea under elevated temperature and humidity. J. agric. Fd Chem., 21, 338-341

Bontoyan, W.R., Looker, J.B., Kaiser, T.E., Giang, P. & Olive, B.M. (1972) Survey of ethylenethiourea in commercial ethylenebisdithiocarbamate formulations. J. Ass. off. analyt. Chem., 55, 923-925

Budnikov, G.K., Toropova, V.F., Ulakhovich, N.A. & Viter, I.P. (1974) Electrochemical behavior of dithiocarbaminates on a mercury electrode. III. Polarographic study of fungicides of dithiocarbaminate type in organic solvents. Zh. analyt. Khim., 29, 1204-1209

California Department of Food and Agriculture (1975) Pesticide Use Report, 1974, Sacramento, pp. 96-98

146

Corneliussen, P.E. (1972) Pesticide residues in total diet samples. VI.
    Pest. Monit. J., 5, 313-330

Engst, R., Schnaak, W. & Lewerenz, H.-J. (1971) Untersuchungen zum Meta-
    bolismus der fungiciden Athylen-bis-dithiocarbamate Maneb, Zinen und
    Nabam. V. Zur Toxikologie der Abbauprodukte. Z. Lebensmittel. Unter-
    such., 146, 91-97

Fishbein, L. (1975) Chromatography of Environmental Hazards, Vol. 3,
    Pesticides, Amsterdam, Elsevier, pp. 676-692

Fishbein, L. & Zielinski, W.L., Jr (1967) Chromatography of carbamates.
    Chromat. Rev., 9, 37-101

Howard, S.F. & Yip, G. (1971) Stability of metallic ethylene bisdithio-
    carbamates in chopped kale. J. Ass. off. analyt. Chem., 54, 1371-1372

IARC (1974) IARC Monographs on the Evaluation of Carcinogenic Risk of
    Chemicals to Man, 7, Some Anti-thyroid and Related Substances, Nitro-
    furans and Industrial Chemicals, Lyon, pp. 45-52

Innes, J.R.M., Ulland, B.M., Valerio, M.G., Petrucelli, L., Fishbein, L.,
    Hart, E.R., Pallotta, A.J., Bates, R.R., Falk, H.L., Gart, J.J.,
    Klein, M., Mitchell, I. & Peters, J. (1969) Bioassay of pesticides
    and industrial chemicals for tumorigenicity in mice: a preliminary
    note. J. nat. Cancer Inst., 42, 1101-1114

Ivanova, L., Sheytanov, M. & Mosheva-Izmirova, N. (1967) Changes in the
    functional state of the thyroid gland upon acute intoxication with
    certain dithiocarbamates, zineb and maneb. C.R. Acad. Bulg. Sci.,
    20, 1011-1013

Ivanova-Chemishanska, L., Markov, D.V. & Dashev, G. (1971) Light and
    electron microscope observations on rat thyroid after administration
    of some dithiocarbamates. Environm. Res., 4, 201-212

Japanese Ministry of Agriculture and Forestry (1975) Noyaku Yoran (Agri-
    cultural Chemicals Annual) 1975, Division of Plant Disease Protection,
    Tokyo, Takeo Endo, pp. 18, 21, 85, 86, 89, 101, 265, 266, 281

Kaloyanova, F., Ivanova, L. & Alexiev, B. (1967) The influence of large
    doses of maneb on the progeny of albino rats. C.R. Acad. Bulg. Sci.,
    20, 1109-1112

Keppel, G.E. (1969) Modification of the carbon disulfide evolution method
    for dithiocarbamate residues. J. Ass. off. analyt. Chem., 52, 162-166

Manske, D.D. & Corneliussen, P.E. (1974) Pesticide residues in total diet
    samples. VII. Pest. Monit. J., 8, 110-114

Marcon, L.V. (1969) The effect of maneb on the embryonal development of
    generative function of rats. Farmakol. i Toksikol., 32, 731-732

McLeod, H.A. & McCully, K.A. (1969) Head space gas procedure for screening food samples for dithiocarbamates pesticide residues. J. Ass. off. analyt. Chem., 52, 1226-1230

Newsome, W.H. (1974) A method for determining ethylenebis(dithiocarbamate) residues on food crops as bis(trifluoroacetamido)ethane. J. agric. Fd Chem., 22, 886-889

NTIS (National Technical Information Service) (1968) Evaluation of Carcinogenic, Teratogenic and Mutagenic Activities of Selected Pesticides and Industrial Chemicals, Vol. 1, Carcinogenic Study, Washington DC, US Department of Commerce

Petrova-Vergieva, T. & Ivanova-Chemishanska, L. (1973) Assessment of the teratogenic activity of dithiocarbamate fungicides. Fd Cosmet. Toxicol., 11, 239-224

Seidler, H., Härtig, M., Schnaak, W. & Engst, R. (1970) Untersuchungen über den Metabolismus einiger Insektizide und Fungizide in der Ratte. II. Verteilung und Abbau von ^{14}C-markiertem Maneb. Die Nahrung, 14, 363-373

Shtenberg, A.I., Kirlich, A.E. & Orlova, N.V. (1969) Toxicological characteristics of maneb used in treatment of food crops. Vop. Pitan., 28, 66-72

Stecher, P.G., ed. (1968) The Merck Index, 8th ed., Rahway, NJ, Merck & Co., p. 642

Stevenson, A. (1972) A simple color spot test for distinguishing between maneb, zineb, mancozeb, and selected mixtures. J. Ass. off. analyt. Chem., 55, 939-941

US Code of Federal Regulations (1974) Protection of Environment, Title 40, part. 180.110, Washington DC, US Government Printing Office, p. 247

US Department of Agriculture (1974) Farmers' Use of Pesticides in 1971, Quantities, Economic Research Service, Agricultural Economic Report No. 252, Washington DC, US Government Printing Office, p. 25

US Environmental Protection Agency (1974) Production, Distribution, Use and Environmental Impact Potential of Selected Pesticides, Office of Pesticide Programs, EPA 54011-74-001, Washington DC, US Government Printing Office, pp. 298-307

Watts, R.R., Storherr, R.W. & Onley, J.H. (1974) Effects of cooking on ethylenebisdithiocarbamate degradation to ethylene thiourea. Bull. environm. Contam. Toxicol., 12, 224-226

WHO (1975a) 1974 Evaluations of some pesticide residues in food. Wld Hlth Org. Pest. Res. Ser., No. 4, pp. 261-263

WHO (1974b) Pesticide residues in food. Report of the 1974 Joint Meeting of the FAO Working Party of Experts on Pesticide Residues and the WHO Expert Committee on Pesticide Residues. Wld Hlth Org. techn. Rep. Ser., No. 574, pp. 26-30

Yip, G., Onley, J.H. & Howard, S.F. (1971) Residues of maneb and ethylene thiourea on field-sprayed lettuce and kale. J. Ass. off. analyt. Chem., 54, 1373-1375

Zweig, G. & Sherma, J. (1972) Dithiocarbamates. In: Zweig, G., ed., Analytical Methods for Pesticides and Plant Growth Regulators, Vol. 6, Gas Chromatographic Analysis, New York, Academic Press, pp. 561-563

METHYL CARBAMATE

1. Chemical and Physical Data

1.1 Synonyms and trade names

Chem. Abstr. Reg. Serial No.: 598-55-0

Chem. Abstr. Name: Carbamic acid, methyl ester

Methylurethan; methylurethane; urethylane

1.2 Chemical formula and molecular weight

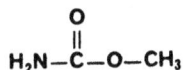

$$\underset{H_2N-\overset{\displaystyle O}{\overset{\|}{C}}-O-CH_3}{}$$

$C_2H_5NO_2$ Mol. wt: 75.1

1.2 Chemical and physical properties of the substance

From Weast (1975), unless otherwise specified

(a) Description: Needles

(b) Boiling-point: 177°C at 760 mm; 82°C at 14 mm

(c) Melting-point: 54°C

(d) Refractive index: n_D^{56} 1.4125

(e) Solubility: Soluble in water (217 parts in 100 at 11°C), ethanol (73 parts in 100 at 15°C) and ether (Prager & Jacobson, 1921)

1.4 Technical products and impurities

No data were available to the Working Group.

2. Production, Use, Occurrence and Analysis

For important background information on this section, see preamble, p. 15.

2.1 Production and use

Methyl carbamate was first prepared by the reaction of cyanogen chloride with methyl alcohol by Echevarria in 1851 (Prager & Jacobson, 1921). It can be made by the reaction of urea with methanol at elevated temperatures using the following catalysts: zinc oxide-phosphoric acid (Vishnyakova *et al.*, 1969), lead oxide (Hata, 1970), aluminosilicate (Vishnyakova *et al.*, 1971) or phosphoric acid (Slater & Culbreth, 1971). It can also be prepared by the reaction of ammonia with methyl chloroformate (Prager & Jacobson, 1921), and this method is believed to have been used commercially.

Commercial production of methyl carbamate was first reported in the US in 1959 (US Tariff Commission, 1960). In 1972, an estimated 350 thousand kg were produced by one manufacturer. In 1973 only two manufacturers reported production (US International Trade Commission, 1975). Annual production of methyl carbamate in Europe is estimated to be 0.75 to 1 million kg.

Methyl carbamate is used as an intermediate in the manufacture of dimethylol methyl carbamate-based resins which are used in the textile industry as durable-press fabric finishes for polyester/cotton blends. Such resins, used principally for treating white cloth, have good crease angle retention, resist acid souring in commercial laundries and do not retain chlorine, if properly cured (Hill, 1967). In Europe, methyl carbamate is also used as a pharmaceutical intermediate.

2.2 Occurrence

Methyl carbamate has been isolated from four *Salsola* species (Karawya *et al.*, 1972).

2.3 Analysis

Methods for the chromatographic analysis of carbamates, including alkyl carbamates, have been reviewed (Fishbein & Zielinski, 1967).

A gas chromatographic method for detection of microgram amounts of methyl carbamate in a mixture of alkyl carbamates after the formation of their trimethylsilyl derivatives has been described (Nery, 1969). Another gas chromatographic method involves the use of an alkali fusion detector,

152

in which the amount of the saponification product, methanol, is determined.
This procedure has been used for determining carbamates, either singly or
in mixtures, at the 0.01-0.1 μM level (Ladas & Ma, 1973).

Colorimetric methods have been used to determine methyl carbamate in
air, at a sensitivity of 20 μg/l (Babina, 1975). Thin-layer and chromatographic methods have also been used for its determination (Karawya *et al.*,
1972; Knappe & Rohdewald, 1966).

3. Biological Data Relevant to the Evaluation of Carcinogenic Risk to Man

3.1 Carcinogenicity and related studies in animals

(a) Subcutaneous administration

Mouse: An unspecified number of random-bred male mice received 3 s.c.
injections of 1 mg/kg bw methyl carbamate at 2-day intervals, and were
observed for 3 months, or 3 s.c. injections of 0.1 mg/kg bw methyl carbamate, and were observed for 6 months. Of those observed for 3 months
(first experiment), 3/29 mice killed had lung adenomas, compared with
3/22 controls and with 23/27 mice given 1 mg/kg bw urethane plus 1 mg/kg bw
methyl carbamate. Of those observed for 6 months (second experiment),
2/26 mice killed had lung adenomas, compared with 0/26 controls and with
6/28 mice given urethane plus methyl carbamate (Yagubov & Suvalova, 1973).

(b) Intraperitoneal administration

Mouse: A group of 46 10-12-week old strain A mice (approximately equal
numbers of each sex) received 13 weekly i.p. injections of 0.5 mg/g recrystallized methyl carbamate in water; the mice were killed 2-3 weeks after
the final injection, when they were 6 months old. Lung adenomas were
found in 16% (mean, 0.19 per mouse), whereas 17% of 141 untreated controls
(mean, 0.18 per mouse) developed these tumours. In two other groups of
43 and 49 mice injected weekly with doses of 1 and 2 mg/g methyl carbamate,
tumour incidences were 9 and 22%, respectively, and average numbers of
tumours per mouse were 0.09 and 0.29. Doses of 3 mg/g induced early deaths
(Larsen, 1947).

A group of 16 7-9-week old male A/He mice was given 12 injections of 5 mg/animal in water over 4 weeks and killed 20 weeks after the end of treatment. Only lung adenoma incidences were reported: 1 lung adenoma was found in 1/16 survivors, compared with 6 lung adenomas in 6/31 mice given the solvent alone and 2 in 2/31 which received no treatment (Shimkin *et al.*, 1969).

(c) Skin application

Mouse: A group of 20 7-9-week old male 'S' mice received 15 weekly cutaneous applications of a 25% solution of methyl carbamate in acetone (total dose, 1.12 g). Three days after the start of the methyl carbamate treatment, 18 weekly applications of croton oil (0.3 ml of a 0.5% solution in acetone) were given. Eighteen mice were still alive at the end of the croton oil treatment, at which time they were killed: 1/18 developed a skin tumour, compared with 1/20 controls given croton oil only. In addition, 7 mice receiving methyl carbamate and croton oil had a total of 12 lung adenomas. No control group killed at the same time is reported (Roe & Salaman, 1955).

(d) Other experimental systems

Subcutaneous injection plus skin promotion: Groups of 40 7-week old male Hall mice were given single s.c. injections of 40 mg methyl carbamate in saline followed 2 weeks later by 24 weekly skin applications of croton oil (0.075% in acetone), or were left untreated. A control group of 80 mice received croton oil only. All animals survived until the end of the croton oil treatment, when observation was discontinued. Two epidermal tumours (unspecified) were found in 1/25 mice receiving methyl carbamate plus croton oil; none were seen in 28 methyl carbamate-injected mice; and 3 occurred in 2/41 mice receiving croton oil only (Pound, 1967).

Injection plus skin promotion: Two groups of 27 and 30 7-week old male Hall mice were given a single injection (route not specified) of 27 mEq/kg bw methyl carbamate. Eighteen hours before treatment those in the second group received an application of 0.25 ml of a 0.075% croton oil solution in acetone over the whole area of the skin of the back. Three weeks later, both groups were given a course of 32 weekly treatments with croton oil, each application consisting of 0.24 ml of an acetone solution, the concentration of which was 0.075% during the first 18 weeks and was then increased to 0.15% for a further 14 weeks. A control group of 90 mice received croton oil alone. The numbers of skin tumour-bearing animals at 36 weeks were 8/86 controls, 8/28 in the first group (P<0.02) and 2/25 (3 tumours) in the second. In animals which died or were killed between 36 and 78 weeks, incidences of skin tumours, hepatomas, liver haemangiomas, lung adenomas and leukaemias were similar in the two experimental groups and in controls receiving croton oil alone (Pound & Lawson, 1976).

3.2 Other relevant biological data

(a) Experimental systems

In mice, the oral LD$_{50}$ of methyl carbamate is 6.2 g/kg bw (Srivalova, 1973).

The rate of metabolism of intraperitoneally injected methyl carbamate is approximately one-half that of ethyl carbamate (urethane) (Boyland & Papadopoulos, 1952; IARC, 1974). Rats injected intraperitoneally with methyl carbamate or the corresponding N-hydroxycarbamate excreted both the carbamate and N-hydroxycarbamate in the urine (Boyland & Nery, 1965).

DNA binding of ^{14}C-ethyl carbamate labelled in either the ethyl or the carbonyl group and of ^{14}C-methyl carbamate labelled in the methyl group has been investigated in mouse liver and kidney. Only ethyl carbamate labelled in the ethyl group binds to liver DNA to a significant extent (Lawson & Pound, 1973). The incorporation of ^{3}H-methyl carbamate into liver-cell RNA has been examined in mice (Williams et al., 1971).

Methyl carbamate did not induce an increase in the number of streptomycin-independent mutations in Escherichia coli (Hemmerly & Demerec, 1955), and no reverse mutations were recorded in Bacillus subtilis (De Giovanni-Donnelly et al., 1967); metabolic activation systems were not used in these tests. An i.p. dose of 200 or 1000 mg/kg caused no increase of dominant lethals in mice (Epstein et al., 1972). In the presence of Aroclor-induced rat liver microsomes, no reverse mutations occurred in Salmonella typhimurium strains TA100, TA98, TA1535 or TA1537 (McCann et al., 1975).

(b) Man

No data were available to the Working Group.

3.3 Case reports and epidemiological studies

No data were available to the Working Group.

4. Comments on Data Reported and Evaluation

4.1 Animal data

Methyl carbamate has been tested for skin and lung tumour induction in mice by subcutaneous and intraperitoneal administration and by skin application. Although no significant carcinogenic effect was observed, no evaluation of carcinogenicity can be made due to the short duration of these experiments. It must be pointed out that in parallel experiments the related chemical, ethyl carbamate, was carcinogenic (IARC, 1974).

4.2 Human data

No case reports or epidemiological studies were available to the Working Group.

5. References

Babina, M.D. (1975) Determination of alkyl carbamates in air. Gig. i Sanit., 7, 76-77

Boyland, E. & Nery, R. (1965) The metabolism of urethane and related compounds. Biochem. J., 94, 198-208

Boyland, E. & Papadopoulos, D. (1952) The metabolism of methyl carbamate. Biochem. J., 52, 267-269

De Giovanni-Donnelly, R., Kolbye, S.M. & DiPaolo, J.A. (1967) Effect of carbamates on *Bacillus subtilis*. Mutation Res., 4, 543-551

Epstein, S.S., Arnold, E., Andrea, J., Bass, W. & Bishop, Y. (1972) Detection of chemical mutagens by the dominant lethal assay in the mouse. Toxicol. appl. Pharmacol., 23, 288-325

Fishbein, L. & Zielinski, W.L., Jr (1967) Chromatography of carbamates. Chromat. Rev., 9, 37-101

Hata, H. (1970) Manufacture of carbamates. Japan Patent 70 23,536, August 7, to Dainippon Ink and Chemicals, Inc. and to Dainippon Ink Research Institute

Hemmerly, J. & Demerec, M. (1955) Tests of chemicals for mutagenicity. Cancer Res., 15, 69-75

Hill, J. (1967) Resin consumption in DP. Textile Industries, 131, 123-126

IARC (1974) IARC Monographs on the Evaluation of Carcinogenic Risk of Chemicals to Man, 7, Some Anti-thyroid and Related Substances, Nitrofurans and Industrial Chemicals, Lyon, pp. 111-140

Karawya, M.S., Wassel, G.M., Baghdadi, H.H. & Ahmed, Z.F. (1972) Isolation of methyl carbamate from four Egyptian *Salsola* species. Phytochemistry, 11, 441-442

Knappe, E. & Rohdewald, I. (1966) Dünnschichtchromatographie von substituierten Harnstoffen und einfachen Urethanen. Z. analyt. Chem., 217, 110-113

Ladas, A.S. & Ma, T.S. (1973) Organic functional group analysis *via* gas chromatography. III. Determination of carbamates by reaction with alkali. Mikrochim. acta (Wien), 853-862

Larsen, C.D. (1947) Evaluation of the carcinogenicity of a series of esters of carbamic acid. J. nat. Cancer Inst., 8, 99-101

Lawson, T.A. & Pound, A.W. (1973) The interaction of carbon-14-labelled alkyl carbamates, labelled in the alkyl and carbonyl positions, with DNA *in vivo*. Chem.-biol. Interact., 6, 99-105

McCann, J., Choi, E., Yamasaki, E. & Ames, B.N. (1975) Detection of carcinogens as mutagens in the *Salmonella*/microsome test: assay of 300 chemicals. Proc. nat. Acad. Sci. (Wash.), 72, 5135-5139

Nery, R. (1969) Gas-chromatographic determination of acetyl and trimethyl-silyl derivatives of alkyl carbamates and their *N*-hydroxy derivatives. Analyst, 94, 130-135

Pound, A.W. (1967) The initiation of skin tumours in mice by homologues and *N*-substituted derivatives of ethyl carbamate. Austr. J. exp. Biol. med. Sci., 45, 507-516

Pound, A.W. & Lawson, T.A. (1976) Carcinogenesis by carbamic acid esters and their binding to DNA. Cancer Res., 36, 1101-1107

Prager, B. & Jacobson, P., eds (1921) Beilsteins Handbuch der organischen Chemie, 4th ed., Vol. 3, Syst. No. 201, p. 21

Roe, F.J.C. & Salaman, M.H. (1955) Further studies on incomplete carcinogenesis: triethylene melamine (T.E.M.), 1,2-benzanthracene and β-propiolactone as initiators of skin tumour formation in the mouse. Brit. J. Cancer, 9, 177-203

Shimkin, M.B., Wieder, R., McDonough, M., Fishbein, L. & Swern, D. (1969) Lung tumor response in strain A mice as a quantitative bioassay of carcinogenic activity of some carbamates and aziridines. Cancer Res., 29, 2184-2190

Slater, J.D. & Culbreth, W.J. (1971) Carbamic ester process and fertilizer values therein. US Patent 3,544,730, January 12, to Kaiser Aluminum and Chemical Co.

Srivalova, T.I. (1973) Toxic and specific action of alkyl carbamates and their binary mixture. Toksikol. Nov. Prom. Khim. Veshchestv., 13, 86-91

US International Trade Commission (1975) Synthetic Organic Chemicals, US Production and Sales, 1973, ITC Publication 728, Washington DC, US Government Printing Office, p. 217

US Tariff Commission (1960) Synthetic Organic Chemicals, US Production and Sales, 1959, Report No. 206, Second Series, Washington DC, US Government Printing Office, p. 160

Vishnyakova, T.P., Paushkin, Y.M., Faltynek, T.A., Golubeva, I.A., Liakumovich, A.G. & Michurov, Y.I. (1969) Synthesis of alkyl carbamates, selective solvents for hydrocarbons. Neftepererab. Neftekhim., 1, 27-29

Vishnyakova, T.P., Paushkin, Y.M., Faltynek, T.A., Golubeva, I.A., Fedorov, V.V. & Shuleiko, G.F. (1971) Synthesis of alkyl carbamates in the presence of an aluminosilicate catalyst. Khim. Tekhnol. Topl. Masel., 16, 10-14

Weast, R.C., ed. (1975) CRC Handbook of Chemistry and Physics, 56th ed., Cleveland, Ohio, Chemical Rubber Co., C-231

Williams, K., Kunz, W., Petersen, K. & Schnieders, B. (1971) Changes in mouse liver RNA induced by ethyl carbamate (urethane) and methyl carbamate. Z. Krebsforsch., 76, 69-82

Yagubov, A.S. & Suvalova, T.I. (1973) Comparative evaluation of the blastomogenic action of a binary mixture of alkylcarbamates and its components. Gig. Tr. Prof. Zabol., 8, 19-22

METHYL SELENAC

1. Chemical and Physical Data

1.1 Synonyms and trade names

Chem. Abstr. Reg. Serial No.: 144-34-3

Chem. Abstr. Name: Tetrakis(dimethylcarbamodithioato-S,S')selenium

Selenium dimethyldithiocarbamate

1.2 Chemical formula and molecular weight

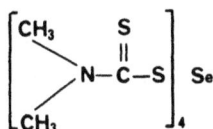

$C_{12}H_{24}N_4S_8Se$ Mol. wt: 559.8

1.3 Chemical and physical properties of the pure substance

No data were available to the Working Group.

1.4 Technical products and impurities

Methyl selenac available commercially in the US has the following specifications: yellow powder; density, 1.58 ± 0.03; melting range, 140-172°C; particle size, 99.9% passes through a 100-mesh screen; selenium content, 13-15%; moisture, 1% max.; ash, 0.75% max. (Anon., 1974). Methyl selenac is also available for rubber processing in a dispersion containing 30% ethylene-propylene rubber binder (Anon., 1975).

2. Production, Use, Occurrence and Analysis

For important background information on this section, see preamble, p. 15.

2.1 Production and use

The usual method for the preparation of water-insoluble dialkyl-dithiocarbamate metal salts is precipitation of the metal salt from an aqueous preparation of the sodium dialkyldithiocarbamate (Shaver, 1968).

Commercial production of methyl selenac was first reported in the US in 1946 (US Tariff Commission, 1948); in 1974, only one manufacturer reported production (US International Trade Commission, 1975). It is not produced commercially in Europe.

Methyl selenac is used in the rubber-processing industry as an accelerator to produce desired physical properties in vulcanized rubber in a shorter curing time and at lower sulphur levels than with conventional accelerators. It is used in compounding heat-resistant natural and synthetic rubbers (Supp & Gibbs, 1974).

According to the US Occupational Safety and Health administration health standards for air contaminants, an employee's exposure to selenium compounds should not exceed 0.2 mg/m³ (as Se) in the workplace air during any eight-hour workshift for a forty-hour work week (US Code of Federal Regulations, 1975). In the USSR, the maximum allowable concentration of selenium compounds in the work environment is 0.1 mg/m³ (Winell, 1975).

2.2 Occurrence

Methyl selenac is not known to occur as a natural product.

2.3 Analysis

Methods for the gas chromatographic analysis of selenium have been reviewed (Young & Christian, 1973). Gas chromatography coupled with a microwave-emission spectrometric detection system has been used for determination of trace amounts of selenium in environmental samples (Talmi & Andren, 1974). Methyl selenac has been determined in rubber additives by both atomic absorption spectrometry and wet analytical determination of selenium (Supp & Gibbs, 1974).

Methods for the chromatographic analysis of carbamates, including thiocarbamates, have been reviewed (Fishbein & Zielinski, 1967). A thin-layer chromatographic-spectrophotofluorimetric method (van Hoof & Heyndrickx,

1973) is suitable for the analysis of a variety of metal dithiocarbamates, although it was not applied to methyl selenac itself.

3. Biological Data Relevant to the Evaluation of Carcinogenic Risk to Man[1]

3.1 Carcinogenicity and related studies in animals

(a) Oral administration

Mouse: Groups of 18 male and 18 female $(C57BL/6xC3H/Anf)F_1$ mice and 18 male and 18 female $(C57BL/6xAKR)F_1$ mice received commercial methyl selenac (m.p. 140-172°C) according to the following schedule: 10 mg/kg bw in gelatine at 7 days of age by stomach tube and the same amount (not adjusted for increasing body weight) daily up to 4 weeks of age; subsequently, the mice were given 34 mg methyl selenac per kg of diet. The dose was the maximum tolerated dose for infant and young mice but not necessarily so for adults. The experiment was terminated when the mice were about 78 weeks of age, at which time 13, 17, 18 and 17 mice in the four groups, respectively, were still alive. Tumour incidences were compared with those observed among 79-90 necropsied mice of each sex and strain, which either had been untreated or had received gelatine only: the incidences were not significantly greater (P>0.05) for any tumour type in any sex-strain subgroup or in the combined sexes of either strain. Tumours were found in 4/17 males and 0/17 females of the first strain and in 1/18 males and 2/17 females of the second strain (5 reticulum-cell sarcomas, 1 hepatoma and 1 renal adenoma) (Innes *et al.*, 1969; NTIS, 1968).

(b) Subcutaneous administration

Mouse: Groups of 18 male and 18 female $(C57BL/6xC3H/Anf)F_1$ mice and 18 male and 18 female $(C57BL/6xAKF)F_1$ mice were given single s.c. injections of 464 mg/kg bw commercial methyl selenac (m.p. 140-172°C) in 0.5% gelatine on the 28th day of life and were observed until they were about 78 weeks of

---

[1]See also the monograph on selenium and selenium compounds (IARC, 1975).

age, at which time 13, 15, 18 and 17 mice in the four groups, respectively, were still alive. Tumour incidences were compared with those in groups of 141, 154, 161 and 157 untreated or vehicle-injected controls that were necropsied. Incidences were not increased (P>0.05) for any tumour type in any sex-strain subgroup or in the combined sexes of either strain (NTIS, 1968) [The Working Group noted that a negative result obtained with a single s.c. injection may not be an adequate basis for discounting carcinogenicity].

3.2 Other relevant biological data

No data were available to the Working Group.

3.3 Case reports and epidemiological studies

No data were available to the Working Group.

4. Comments on Data Reported and Evaluation

4.1 Animal data

Methyl selenac has been tested by oral administration and by single s.c. injection in two strains of mice. Although no carcinogenic effect was observed in these tests, the available data are insufficient to allow an evaluation of the carcinogenicity of this compound.

4.2 Human data

No case reports or epidemiological studies were available to the Working Group.

5. References

Anon. (1974) Methyl Selenac®, New York, R.T. Vanderbilt Co.

Anon. (1975) Materials and Compounding Ingredients for Rubber, New York, Bill Communications, pp. 47-48

Fishbein, L. & Zielinski, W.L., Jr (1967) Chromatography of carbamates. Chromat. Rev., 9, 37-101

van Hoof, F. & Heyndrickx, A. (1973) Thin layer chromatographic-spectrophotofluorimetric methods for the determination of dithio- and thiolcarbamates after hydrolysis and coupling with NBD-Cl. Ghent. Rijksuniv. Fac. Landbl. Med., 38, 911-916

IARC (1975) IARC monographs on the Evaluation of Carcinogenic Risk of Chemicals to Man, 9, Some Aziridines, N-, S- and O-Mustards and Selenium, Lyon, pp. 250-251

Innes, J.R.M., Ulland, B.M., Valerio, M.G., Petrucelli, L., Fishbein, L., Hart, E.R., Pallotta, A.J., Bates, R.R., Falk, H.L., Gart, J.J., Klein, M., Mitchell, I. & Peters, J. (1969) Bioassay of pesticides and industrial chemicals for tumorigenicity in mice: a preliminary note. J. nat. Cancer Inst., 42, 1101-1114

NTIS (National Technical Information Service) (1968) Evaluation of Carcinogenic, Teratogenic and Mutagenic Activities of Selected Pesticides and Industrial Chemicals, Vol. 1, Carcinogenic Study, Washington DC, US Department of Commerce

Shaver, F.W. (1968) Rubber chemicals. In: Kirk, R.E. & Othmer, D.F., eds, Encyclopedia of Chemical Technology, 2nd ed., Vol. 17, New York, John Wiley & Sons, pp. 513-514

Supp, G.R. & Gibbs, I. (1974) The determination of selenium and tellurium in organic accelerators used in the vulcanization process for natural and synthetic rubbers by atomic absorption spectrometry. Atomic Absorption Newslett., 13, 71-73

Talmi, Y. & Andren, A.W. (1974) Determination of selenium in environmental samples using gas chromatography with a microwave emission spectrometric detection system. Analyt. Chem., 46, 2122-2126

US Code of Federal Regulations (1975) Air Contaminants, Title 29, part. 1910.1000, Washington DC, US Government Printing Office, pp. 59, 61

US International Trade Commission (1975) Synthetic Organic Chemicals, US Production and Sales of Rubber-Processing Chemicals, 1974 Preliminary, Washington DC, US Government Printing Office, p. 8

US Tariff Commission (1948) Synthetic Organic Chemicals, US Production and Sales, 1946, Report No. 159, Second Series, Washington DC, US Government Printing Office, p. 123, 155

Winell, M.A. (1975) An international comparison of hygienic standards for chemicals in the work environment. Ambio, 4, 34-36

Young, J.W. & Christian, G.D. (1973) Gas-chromatographic determination of selenium. Analyt. chim. acta, 65, 127-138

MONURON

1. Chemical and Physical Data

1.1 Synonyms and trade names

Chem. Abstr. Reg. Serial No.: 150-68-5

Chem. Abstr. Name: *N'*-(4-Chlorophenyl)-*N*,*N*-dimethylurea

1-*para*-Chlorophenyl-3,3-dimethylurea; 3-(4-chlorophenyl)-1,1-dimethylurea; 3'-(4'-chlorophenyl)-1,1-dimethylurea; 3-*para*-chlorophenyl-1,1-dimethylurea; *N*-(4-chlorophenyl)-*N'*,*N'*-dimethylurea; *N*-*para*-chlorophenyl-*N'*,*N'*-dimethylurea; CMU; 1,1-dimethyl-3-(*para*-chlorophenyl)urea; *N*,*N*-dimethyl-*N'*-(4-chlorophenyl)urea

Karmex Monuron Herbicide; Karmex W. Monuron Herbicide; Monurex; Monurox; Monuruon; Monuuron; Telvar; Telvar Monuron Weedkiller; Telvar W. Monuron Weedkiller

1.2 Chemical formula and molecular weight

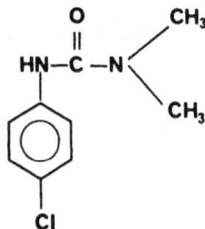

$$C_9H_{11}ClN_2O \qquad \text{Mol. wt: } 198.6$$

1.3 Chemical and physical properties of the substance

From Weast (1975), unless otherwise specified

(a) Description: Platelets

(b) Melting-point: 170.5-171.5°C

(c) Spectroscopy data: λ_{max} = 247 nm (Stecher, 1968); for infra-red and mass spectral data, see Grasselli (1973)

(d) Solubility: Very slightly soluble in water, in hydrocarbon solvents and in No. 3 diesel oil (Stecher, 1968); moderately soluble in methanol, ethanol and acetone

(e) Volatility: Vapour pressure is 5×10^{-7} mm at $25^\circ C$ and 178×10^{-5} mm at $100^\circ C$ (Stecher, 1968).

(f) Stability: Negligible hydrolysis at room temperatures in neutral solutions (Association of American Pesticide Control Officials, Inc., 1962)

1.4 Technical products and impurities

Monuron is available in the US as a technical grade product, as a wettable powder containing about 80% of the chemical and as granular formulations containing 2.4-8%. Granular formulations containing both monuron and trichloroacetic acid are also available, with several concentrations of each active ingredient (US Environmental Protection Agency, 1975).

2. Production, Use, Occurrence and Analysis

For important background information on this section, see preamble, p. 15. A review on monuron has been published (US Environmental Protection Agency, 1975).

2.1 Production and use

Eight methods for the synthesis of monuron have been reported (US Environmental Protection Agency, 1975); the method used commercially is believed to be the reaction of *para*-chloroaniline with phosgene and subsequently with dimethylamine (Plimmer, 1970).

Monuron was first produced commercially in the US in 1951 (US Tariff Commission, 1952). US production in 1973 was estimated to be 230-400 thousand kg; somewhat larger quantities are believed to have been produced in earlier years when wider use was permitted in the US and a lesser number of competitive products existed. US imports in 1973 were 65 thousand kg, and exports were about 45 thousand kg (US Environmental Protection Agency, 1975).

The only known use of monuron is as a broad-spectrum herbicide for the control of many grasses and herbaceous weeds on non-cropland areas, such as rights-of-way, industrial sites and drainage ditch banks. In the past, monuron was registered in the US for selective control of weeds in several crops, and monuron residues of 1-7 mg/kg were tolerated on a variety of fruits and vegetables. As of July 1973, however, monuron is no longer registered for use on any agricultural crop (US Environmental Protection Agency, 1975).

2.2 Occurrence

Monuron is not known to occur as a natural product.

When it was applied at rates formerly used on crops, phytotoxic concentrations disappeared from the soil within one year. When applied at non-selective rates for total vegetation control, e.g., on rights-of-way, it retains its phytotoxic activity for several seasons. Larger applications of monuron (20 to 200 kg/hectare) have required up to 3 years to dissipate (US Environmental Protection Agency, 1975).

In one investigation of the persistence of monuron in river water, acetone solutions of monuron were injected into water samples which were exposed to natural and artificial light at room temperature. By the end of 1 week, 40% of the monuron remained; at 2 weeks, 30%; at 4 weeks, 20%; and at 8 weeks, 0% (US Environmental Protection Agency, 1975).

2.3 Analysis

Methods for the determination of monuron have been reviewed (Lowen *et al.*, 1964; Zweig & Sherma, 1972), and several other reviews have dealt with analytical methods for pesticides structurally related to this material (Fishbein, 1975; Sherma, 1973). A review has also been made of methods of mass spectrometry for a variety of pesticides, including monuron (Safe & Hutzinger, 1973).

Gas chromatography has been used to determine monuron and its hydrolosis products (Buser & Grolimund, 1974; Gutenmann & Lisk, 1964; Lawrence & Laver, 1974; Lichtenberg, 1975). Geike (1973) described a thin-layer chromatographic screening test for phenylurea herbicides that inhibit certain enzymic activities.

A rapid bioluminescence method capable of determining low concentrations of photosynthesis-inhibiting herbicides, such as monuron, in water and soil has been described by Tchan *et al.* (1975).

3. Biological Data Relevant to the Evaluation
of Carcinogenic Risk to Man

3.1 Carcinogenicity and related studies in animals

(a) Oral administration

Mouse: Groups of 18 male and 18 female (C57BL/6xC3H/Anf)F_1 mice and 18 male and 18 female (C57BL/6xAKR)F_1 mice received commercial monuron (95% pure) according to the following schedule: 215 mg/kg bw in 0.5% gelatine at 7 days of age by stomach tube and the same amount (not adjusted for increasing body weight) daily up to 4 weeks of age; subsequently, the mice were given 517 mg per kg of diet. The dose was the maximum tolerated dose for infant and young mice but not necessarily so for adults. The experiment was terminated when the mice were about 78 weeks of age, at which time 15, 18, 16 and 17 mice in the four groups, respectively, were still alive. Tumour incidences were compared with those in 79-90 necropsied mice of each sex and strain, which either had been untreated or had received gelatine only. Tumours occurred in 7/15 necropsied males (2 reticulum-cell sarcomas, 2 lung adenomas, 3 hepatomas) and in 0/18 necropsied females of the first strain, and in 6/16 necropsied males (6 lung adenomas) and in 3/17 necropsied females (1 reticulum-cell sarcoma and 2 lung adenomas) of the second strain. Tumour incidences were significantly different only for lung adenomas in males of the second strain (6/16 compared with 9/90) [P<0.01] (Innes *et al.*, 1969; NTIS, 1968).

Groups of 25 random-bred and 25 C57BL mice (sex unspecified) were given 6 mg/animal monuron in milk by stomach tube weekly for 13 months, at which time the 23 and 25 survivors were killed. A total of 13 tumours occurred in 13 random-bred mice, comprising 1 stomach adenocarcinoma, 4 hepatomas, 4 hepatocellular carcinomas, 2 lung tumours and 2 malignant kidney tumours. Of the 25 C57BL mice, 7 had tumours, comprising 1 lymphoma of the intestine, 2 hepatomas, 2 liver-cell carcinomas, 1 lung tumour and 1 malignant kidney tumour. No tumours occurred in an equal number of untreated random-bred controls; one hepatoma occurred among C57BL controls; however, survival rates among controls were not reported (Rubenchik et al., 1970).

Rat: Four groups of 30 male and 30 female 4-week old albino rats (Rochester, ex-Wistar) were fed diets containing 0 (control), 0.0025, 0.025 or 0.25% monuron for up to 2 years, at which time 10-30% were still alive. Twenty-four tumours (mainly lymphomas and mammary fibroadenomas) occurred in the groups killed at 2 years, and about 30 rats died with tumours before 2 years. The total tumour incidence was reported to be within the range of that in control rats of that colony (Hodge et al., 1958) [Incomplete reporting of data makes evaluation of this experiment difficult].

A group of 50 random-bred male rats was given 450 mg/kg monuron in the food daily for 18 months and observed for a further 9 months, at which time 32 treated and 30 control rats were still alive. Tumours occurred in 14 rats and included 2 stomach tumours, 1 malignant tumour of the intestine, 1 hepatoma, 2 liver-cell carcinomas, 2 alveolar carcinomas, 4 small-cell carcinomas of the lung and 2 seminomas. The first tumour appeared after 18 weeks. No tumours were reported to have occurred in 50 control rats (Rubenchik et al., 1970) [The absence of tumours in controls was considered to be unusual].

(b) Subcutaneous administration

Mouse: Groups of 18 male and 18 female (C57BL/6xC3H/Anf)F_1 mice and 18 male and 18 female (C57BL/6xAKR)F_1 mice were given single s.c. injections of 100 mg/kg bw monuron (95% pure) in 0.5% gelatine on the 28th day of life and were observed until they were about 78 weeks of age, at which time 15, 18, 18 and 16 mice in the four groups, respectively, were still alive. Tumour incidences were compared with those in groups of 141, 154, 161 and 157 untreated or vehicle-injected controls that were necropsied. Incidences were not increased (P>0.05) for any tumour type in any sex-strain subgroup or in the combined sexes of either strain (NTIS, 1968) [The Working Group noted that a negative result obtained with a single s.c. injection may not be an adequate basis for discounting carcinogenicity].

3.2 Other relevant biological data

(a) Experimental systems

The oral LD$_{50}$ in rats ranged from 1480 to 3700 mg/kg bw (Ben-Dyke et al., 1970). No toxic effects were observed in rats following oral administration of 25 mg/kg bw/day for 2 years; doses 10 times higher produced slight toxic effects (Hodge et al., 1958).

In rats given 875 mg/kg bw orally, peak blood concentrations occurred 2 hours after dosing; thereafter, the compound was distributed evenly throughout the body. Monuron-related material was excreted in the urine and secreted into the milk of lactating animals. After administration of 175 mg/kg bw/day for 60 days or of 0.1-20.0 mg/kg bw/day for 6 months, tissue retention of monuron-related substances occurred in the lungs > heart > liver, brain and kidneys > milk, bone-marrow and thyroid gland (Fridman, 1968).

In mammals, monuron is metabolized (i) by oxidative N-demethylation, (ii) by hydroxylation of the aromatic nucleus and (iii) by fission of the urea residue to give chloroaniline derivatives (Ernst, 1969; Ernst & Böhme, 1965). The principal urinary metabolites of monuron (1) (Scheme 1) in rats are N-(4-chlorophenyl)-N'-methylurea (2), N-(4-chlorophenyl)urea (3) (14.5% of the dose), N-(2-hydroxy-4-chlorophenyl)-N',N'-dimethylurea (4), N-(2-hydroxy-4-chlorophenyl)-N'-methylurea (5) (1.5%), N-(2-hydroxy-4-chlorophenyl)urea (6) (6.5%), 2-acetamino-5-chlorophenol (7) and N-(3-hydroxy-4-chlorophenyl)urea (8) (2.2%).

The yields of the various metabolites indicate that hydroxylation favours the 2-position rather than the 3-position. Phenolic metabolites were excreted in the urine as conjugates. 4-Chloro-2-hydroxyaniline was excreted as the N-acetyl compound (7) (Ernst, 1969; Ernst & Böhme, 1965).

(b) Man

No data were available to the Working Group.

3.3 Case reports and epidemiological studies

No data were available to the Working Group.

SCHEME 1

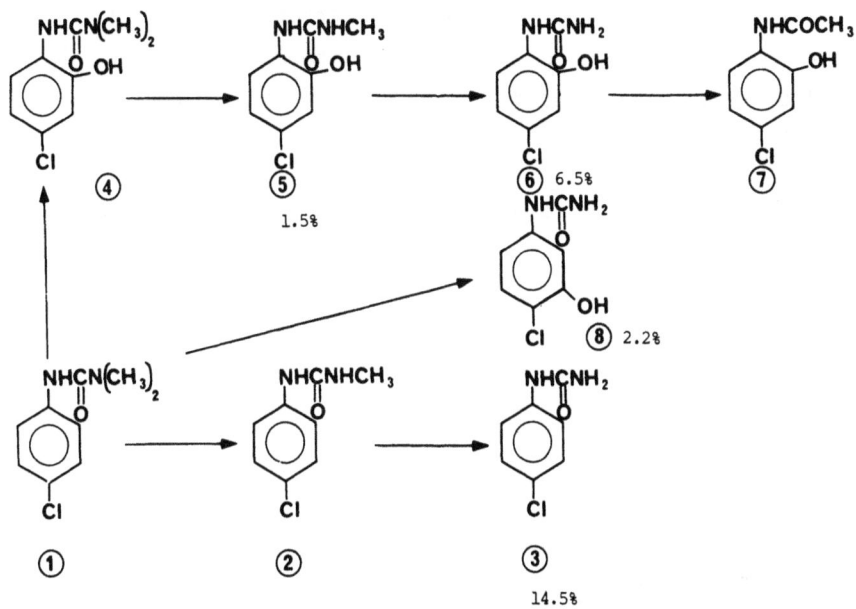

4. Comments on Data Reported and Evaluation

4.1 Animal data

Monuron has been tested in mice and rats by oral administration and in mice by single subcutaneous injection. In one study by oral administration in mice, an increased incidence of lung tumours was observed in males of one of two strains. In a further study in mice, an increased incidence of liver tumours was observed, but survival rates in controls were not reported. In one study by oral administration in male rats, tumours were observed at various sites; none were observed in concurrent controls. The available data suggest that monuron is carcinogenic.

4.2 Human data

No case reports or epidemiological studies were available to the Working Group.

5. References

Association of American Pesticide Control Officials, Inc. (1962) Pesticide Chemicals Official Compendium, Box HH, University P.O., College Park, Maryland, p. 211

Ben-Dyke, R., Sanderson, D.M. & Noakes, D.N. (1970) Acute toxicity data for pesticides (1970). Wld Rev. Pest. Control, 9, 119-127

Buser, H. & Grolimund, K. (1974) Direct determination of N'-phenyl urea derivatives in herbicide technical products and formulations, using gas-liquid chromatography. J. Ass. off. analyt. Chem., 57, 1294-1299

Ernst, W. (1969) Metabolism of substituted dinitrophenols and ureas in mammals and methods for the isolation and identification of metabolites. J. Suid-Afrik. chem. Inst., 22, S79-S88

Ernst, W. & Böhme, C. (1965) Über den Stoffwechsel von Harnstoff-Herbiciden in der Ratte. I. Monuron und Aresin. Fd Cosmet. Toxicol., 3, 789-796

Fishbein, L. (1975) Chromatography of Environmental Hazards, Vol. 3, Pesticides, Amsterdam, Elsevier, pp. 690-732

Fridman, E.B. (1968) Distribution and accumulation of monuron in animals, and methods of its excretion. Zdravookhr. Turkm., 12, 25-27

Geike, F. (1973) Thin-layer chromatographic screening test for the detection of inhibiting properties of phenylurea herbicides on certain enzymes. J. Chromat., 87, 199-210

Grasselli, J.G., ed. (1973) Atlas of Spectral Data and Physical Constants for Organic Compounds, Cleveland, Ohio, Chemical Rubber Co., p. B-983

Gutenmann, W.H. & Lisk, D.J. (1964) Electron affinity residue determination of CIPC, monuron, diuron, and linuron by direct hydrolysis and bromination. J. agric. Fd Chem., 12, 46-48

Hodge, H.C., Maynard, E.A., Downs, W.L. & Coye, R.D. (1958) Chronic toxicity of 3-(p-chlorophenyl)-1,1-dimethylurea (monuron). Arch. industr. Hlth, 17, 45-47

Innes, J.R.M., Ulland, B.M., Valerio, M.G., Petrucelli, L., Fishbein, L., Hart, E.R., Pallotta, A.J., Bates, R.R., Falk, H.L., Gart, J.J., Klein, M., Mitchell, I. & Peters, J. (1969) Bioassay of pesticides and industrial chemicals for tumorigenicity in mice: a preliminary note. J. nat. Cancer Inst., 42, 1101-1114

Lawrence, J.F. & Laver, G.W. (1974) Analysis of carbamate and urea herbicides in foods, using fluorogenic labeling. J. Ass. off. analyt. Chem., 57, 1022-1025

Lichtenberg, J.J. (1975) Methods for the determination of specific organic pollutants in water and waste water. Inst. Electrical Electronics Engineers Trans. Nuclear Sci., NS-22, 874-891

Lowen, W.K., Bleidner, W.E., Kirkland, J.J. & Pease, H.L. (1964) Monuron, Diuron, and Neburon. In: Zweig, G., ed., Analytical Methods for Pesticides, Plant Growth Regulators and Food Additives, Vol. 4, Herbicides, New York, Academic Press, pp. 157-170

NTIS (National Technical Information Service) (1968) Evaluation of Carcinogenic, Teratogenic and Mutagenic Activities of Selected Pesticides and Industrial Chemicals, Vol. 1, Carcinogenic Study, Washington DC, US Department of Commerce

Plimmer, J.R. (1970) Weed killers. In: Kirk, R.E. & Othmer, D.F., eds, Encyclopedia of Chemical Technology, 2nd ed., Vol. 22, New York, John Wiley & Sons, pp. 188-191

Rubenchik, B.L., Botsman, N.E. & Gorbanj, G.P. (1970) On carcinogenic effect of herbicide monuron. Vop. Onkol., 16, 51-53

Safe, S. & Hutzinger, O. (1973) Mass Spectrometry of Pesticides and Pollutants, Cleveland, Ohio, Chemical Rubber Co., pp. 147-151

Sherma, J. (1973) Chromatographic analysis of pesticide residues. CRC Crit. Rev. analyt. Chem., 3, 299-354

Stecher, P.G., ed. (1968) The Merck Index, 8th ed., Rahway, NJ, Merck & Co., pp. 700-701

Tchan, Y.T., Roseby, J.E. & Funnell, G.R. (1975) A new rapid specific bioassay method for photosynthesis inhibiting herbicides. Soil Biol. Biochem., 7, 39-44

US Environmental Protection Agency (1975) Initial Scientific and Mini-economic Review of Monuron. Substitute Chemical Program, EPA-540/1-75-028, Washington DC, US Department of Commerce, pp. 2, 5, 21, 92-93, 98-101

US Tariff Commission (1952) Synthetic Organic Chemicals, US Production and Sales, 1951, Report No. 175, Second Series, Washington DC, US Government Printing Office, p. 135

Weast, R.C., ed. (1975) CRC Handbook of Chemistry and Physics, 56th ed., Cleveland, Ohio, Chemical Rubber Co., p. C531

Zweig, G. & Sherma, J. (1972) Monuron, Diuron, and Neburon. In: Zweig, G., ed., Analytical Methods for Pesticides, Plant Growth Regulators and Food Additives, Vol. 6, Gas chromatographic analysis, New York, Academic Press, pp. 664-666

PHENICARBAZIDE

1. Chemical and Physical Data

1.1 Synonyms and trade names

Chem. Abstr. Reg. Serial No.: 39538-93-7

Chem. Abstr. Name: 2-Phenylhydrazinecarboxamide

1-Carbamoyl-2-phenylhydrazine; 1-carbamyl-2-phenylhydrazine; 2-phenyldiazenecarboxamide; 2-phenylhydrazide, carbamic acid; 1-phenylhydrazine carboxamide; phenylsemicarbazide; 1-phenylsemi-carbazide

CPH; Cryogenine; Kryogenin

1.2 Chemical formula and molecular weight

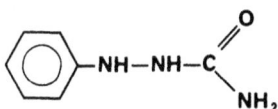

$C_7H_9N_3O$ Mol. wt: 151.2

1.3 Chemical and physical properties of the substance

From Stecher (1968), unless otherwise specified

(a) Description: Leaflets from water

(b) Melting-point: $172^{\circ}C$

(c) Spectroscopy data: λ_{max} = 282 and 233 nm in methanol (Grasselli, 1973); for infra-red spectral data, see Grasselli (1973)

(d) Solubility: Very soluble in hot water, ethanol, methanol and acetone; slightly soluble in cold water, ethyl ether, benzene and ligroin

1.4 Technical products and impurities

No data were available to the Working Group.

2. Production, Use, Occurrence and Analysis

For important background information on this section, see preamble, p. 15.

2.1 Production and use

Preparation of phenicarbazide was first reported in 1893 by Wildman, who synthesized it by reacting an aqueous solution of phenylhydrazine acetate with potassium cyanate (Stecher, 1968). It can also be prepared by adding urea to an aqueous solution of phenylhydrazine (Andraca, 1941).

No indication was found that phenicarbazide is produced in commercial quantities in the US, although it is produced by one manufacturer for research purposes. It was estimated that 5 thousand kg were produced in Italy in 1975.

Phenicarbazide has been tested clinically as an antipyretic and as a neuroleptic agent (Nucifora & Malone, 1971) and has been described in patents for use as an aldehyde polymerization catalyst and stabilizer for vinyl compounds; however, no evidence was found that it is used commercially for these purposes.

2.2 Occurrence

Phenicarbazide is not known to occur as a natural product.

2.3 Analysis

No analytical methods suitable for the determination of phenicarbazide in environmental samples were available to the Working Group.

3.   Biological Data Relevant to the Evaluation
of Carcinogenic Risk to Man[1]

3.1 Carcinogenicity and related studies in animals

Oral administration

Mouse: Commercial phenicarbazide (m.p. 174-175°C) was administered
for lifespan to 50 7-week old female and 50 7-week old male Swiss mice
as a 0.25% solution in the drinking-water. The daily intake was 20.4 mg/
female and 25 mg/male. Lifespan of treated animals was shortened, particularly for males: 11 females and 5 males lived to 80 weeks of age
versus 71/100 and 65/100 controls. In treated animals, 205 lung tumours
were found in 39/50 females (30 with 126 adenomas; 9 with 18 adenocarcinomas and 61 adenomas) and 152 in 33/49 males (28 with 108 adenomas;
5 with 8 adenocarcinomas and 36 adenomas), compared with 31 in 21/99
untreated females (17 with 23 adenomas; 3 with 5 adenocarcinomas; 1
with 1 adenoma and 2 adenocarcinomas) and 35 in 23/99 untreated males
(10 with 12 adenomas; 8 with 11 adenocarcinomas; 5 with 6 adenomas and
6 adenocarcinomas). Average ages at death in mice with lung tumours
were 73 and 64 weeks in treated females and males, respectively, and
95 and 92 weeks in control females and males, respectively. Angiomas
or angiosarcomas were found in the livers of 12/99 treated mice and of
9/198 controls (P<0.02). Tumours occurred at other sites in low incidences (Toth & Shimizu, 1974).

3.2 Other relevant biological data

No data were available to the Working Group.

3.3 Case reports and epidemiological studies

No data were available to the Working Group.

---

[1]Phenicarbazide is a hydrazine derivative. For a discussion of
hydrazine and related substances, see IARC (1974).

4. Comments on Data Reported and Evaluation[1]

4.1 Animal data

Phenicarbazide is carcinogenic in mice when administered orally, the only species and route investigated. It produced lung tumours and angiomas and/or angiosarcomas in the liver.

4.2 Human data

No case reports or epidemiological studies were available to the Working Group.

---

[1]See also the section, 'Animal data in relation to the evaluation of risk to man' in the introduction to this volume, p. 13.

5. References

Andraca, A. (1941) Study and synthesis of phenylsemicarbazide. An. quim. farm., 15-26

Grasselli, J.G., ed. (1973) Atlas of Spectral Data and Physical Constants for Organic Compounds, Cleveland, Ohio, Chemical Rubber Co., p. B-891

IARC (1974) IARC Monographs on the Evaluation of Carcinogenic Risk of Chemicals to Man, 4, Some Aromatic Amines, Hydrazine and Related Substances, N-Nitroso Compounds and Miscellaneous Alkylating Agents, Lyon, pp. 127-136

Nucifora, T.L. & Malone, M.H. (1971) Comparative psychopharmacologic investigation of cryogenine, certain nonsteroid antiinflammatory compounds, lupine alkaloids, and cyproheptadine. Arch. int. Pharmacodyn. Ther., 191, 345-356

Stecher, P.G., ed. (1968) The Merck Index, 8th ed., Rahway, NJ, Merck & Co., p. 808

Toth, B. & Shimizu, H. (1974) 1-Carbamyl-2-phenylhydrazine tumorigenesis in Swiss mice. Morphology of lung adenomas. J. nat. Cancer Inst., 52, 241-251

POTASSIUM BIS(2-HYDROXYETHYL)DITHIOCARBAMATE

1. Chemical and Physical Data

1.1 Synonyms and trade names

Chem. Abstr. Reg. Serial No.: 23746-34-1

Chem. Abstr. Name: Bis(2-hydroxyethyl)carbamodithioic acid, monopotassium salt

Bis(2-hydroxyethyl)dithiocarbamic acid, monopotassium salt

1.2 Chemical formula and molecular weight

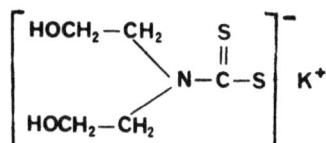

$$\left[\begin{array}{c} HOCH_2-CH_2 \\ \\ HOCH_2-CH_2 \end{array} \diagdown N-\overset{\overset{\displaystyle S}{\|}}{C}-S \right]^{-} K^{+}$$

$$C_5H_{10}KNO_2S_2 \qquad \text{Mol. wt: } 219.4$$

1.3 Chemical and physical properties of the pure substance

No data were available to the Working Group.

1.4 Technical products and impurities

No data were available to the Working Group.

2. Production, Use, Occurrence and Analysis

For important background information on this section, see preamble, p. 15.

2.1 Production and use

Potassium bis(2-hydroxyethyl)dithiocarbamate can be prepared by the addition of carbon disulphide to an aqueous solution of diethanolamine and potassium hydroxide. No indication has been found that it is produced in commercial quantities in the US or Europe. Two US companies offer it for research purposes (Anon., 1975).

Potassium bis(2-hydroxyethyl)dithiocarbamate can be used as an analytical reagent for the quantitative determination of mercury, palladium (Usatenko *et al.*, 1971), gold (Garus *et al.*, 1968), copper, cobalt and nickel (Balatre & Pinkas, 1961; Pinkas, 1960).

2.2 Occurrence

Potassium bis(2-hydroxyethyl)dithiocarbamate is not known to occur as a natural product.

2.3 Analysis

No analytical methods suitable for the determination of potassium bis(2-hydroxyethyl)dithiocarbamate in environmental samples were available to the Working Group. A thin-layer chromatographic-spectrofluorimetric method (van Hoof & Heyndrickx, 1973) is suitable for the analysis of a variety of metal dithiocarbamates, although it was not applied to potassium bis(2-hydroxyethyl)dithiocarbamate itself.

3. Biological Data Relevant to the Evaluation of Carcinogenic Risk to Man

3.1 Carcinogenicity and related studies in animals

(a) Oral administration

Mouse: Groups of 18 male and 18 female (C57BL/6xC3H/Anf)F_1 mice and 18 male and 18 female (C57BL/6xAKR)F_1 mice received commercial potassium bis(2-hydroxyethyl)dithiocarbamate (purity unspecified) according to the following schedule: 464 mg/kg bw in gelatine at 7 days of age by stomach tube and the same amount (not adjusted for increasing body weight) daily up to 4 weeks of age; subsequently, the mice were given 1112 mg potassium bis(2-hydroxyethyl)dithiocarbamate per kg of diet. The dose was the maximum tolerated dose for infant and young mice but not necessarily so for adults. The experiment was terminated when the mice were about 78 weeks of age, at which time 14, 17, 15 and 16 mice in the four groups, respectively, were still alive. Tumour incidences were compared with those observed among 79-90 necropsied mice of each sex and strain, which either had been untreated or had received gelatine only. Hepatomas were found in 13/16 male and 12/18 female (C57BL/6xC3H/Anf)F$_1$ mice, compared with 8/79 and 0/87 controls, and in 13/17 male and 3/16 female (C57BL/6x AKR)F$_1$ mice, compared with 5/90 and 1/82 controls. Incidences of lung adenomas and malignant lymphomas were not greater than those in controls (Innes *et al.*, 1969; NTIS, 1968).

Rat: Results of a 2-year feeding study with potassium bis(2-hydroxy-ethyl)dithiocarbamate in Charles River CD rats have been reported briefly (Ulland *et al.*, 1973) [The inadequate reporting does not allow an evaluation of this experiment].

(b) Subcutaneous administration

Mouse: Groups of 18 male and 18 female (C57BL/6xC3H/Anf)F$_1$ mice and 18 male and 18 female (C57BL/6xAKR)F$_1$ mice were given single s.c. injections of 464 mg/kg bw commercial potassium bis(2-hydroxyethyl)dithiocarbamate (purity unspecified) in dimethyl sulphoxide on the 28th day of life and were observed until they were about 78 weeks of age, at which time 15, 15, 17 and 18 mice in the four groups, respectively, were still alive. Tumour incidences were compared with those in groups of 141, 154, 161 and 157 untreated or vehicle-injected controls that were necropsied. Incidences were not increased (P>0.05) for any tumour type in any sex-strain subgroup or in the combined sexes of either strain (NTIS, 1968) [The Working Group noted that a negative result obtained with a single s.c. injection may not be an adequate basis for discounting carcinogenicity].

3.2 Other relevant biological data

No data were available to the Working Group.

3.3 Case reports and epidemiological studies

No data were available to the Working Group.

4. Comments on Data Reported and Evaluation[1]

4.1 Animal data

Potassium bis(2-hydroxyethyl)dithiocarbamate is carcinogenic in mice after its oral administration: it induced liver-cell tumours in males of two strains and in females of one strain.

4.2 Human data

No case reports or epidemiological studies were available to the Working Group.

_____

[1]See also the section, 'Animal data in relation to the evaluation of risk to man' in the introduction to this volume, p. 13.

5. References

Anon. (1975) Chem. Sources-USA, Flemington, NJ, Directories Publishing
    Co., p. 106

Balatre, P. & Pinkas, M. (1961) Simultaneous colorimetric determination
    of copper and nickel or copper and cobalt by using potassium bis(hy-
    droxyethyl)dithiocarbamate. Chim. analyt., 43, 433-438

Garus, Z.F., Tulyupa, F.M. & Usatenko, Y.I. (1968) Potassium bis(2-hydroxy-
    ethyl)dithiocarbamate, an amperometric reagent for determining small
    amounts of gold (III). Opred. Mikroprimesei, 2, 72-77

van Hoof, F. & Heyndrickx, A. (1973) Thin layer chromatographic-spectro-
    photophuorimetric methods for the determination of dithio- and
    thiolcarbamates after hydrolysis and coupling with NBD-Cl. Ghent.
    Rijksuniv. Fac. Landbl. Med., 38, 911-916

Innes, J.R.M., Ulland, B.M., Valerio, M.G., Petrucelli, L., Fishbein, L.,
    Hart, E.R., Pallotta, A.J., Bates, R.R., Falk, H.L., Gart, J.J.,
    Klein, M., Mitchell, I. & Peters, J. (1969) Bioassay of pesticides
    and industrial chemicals for tumorigenicity in mice: a preliminary
    note. J. nat. Cancer Inst., 42, 1101-1114

NTIS (National Technical Information Service) (1968) Evaluation of Carcino-
    genic, Teratogenic and Mutagenic Activities of Selected Pesticides and
    Industrial Chemicals, Vol. 1, Carcinogenic Study, Washington DC, US
    Department of Commerce

Pinkas, M. (1960) The use of potassium bis(hydroxyethyl)dithiocarbamate in
    the colorimetric determination of copper, cobalt, and nickel. Bull.
    Soc. pharm. Lille, 3, 93-97

Ulland, B., Weisburger, E.K. & Weisburger, J.H. (1973) Chronic toxicity
    and carcinogenicity of industrial chemicals and pesticides. Toxicol.
    appl. Pharmacol., 25, 446

Usatenko, Y.I., Tulyupa, F.M. & Tkacheva, L.M. (1971) Use of potassium
    N,N-bis(2-hydroxyethyl)dithiocarbamate for the amperometric deter-
    mination of mercury and palladium. Khim. Tekhnol. (Kharkov), 18,
    150-154

PROPHAM

1. Chemical and Physical Data

1.1 Synonyms and trade names

Chem. Abstr. Reg. Serial No.: 122-42-9

Chem. Abstr. Name: Phenylcarbamic acid, 1-methylethyl ester

Carbanilic acid isopropyl ester; IFC; INPC; IPC; Iso. PPC.; isopropyl carbanilate; isopropyl carbanilic acid ester; isopropyl phenylcarbamate; isopropyl N-phenylcarbamate; O-isopropyl N-phenyl carbamate; N-phenylcarbamic acid isopropyl ester; N-phenyl isopropyl carbamate

Ban-Hoe; Beet-Kleen; Chem-Hoe; IFK; Triherbide-IPC; Tuberite; Y 2

1.2 Chemical formula and molecular weight

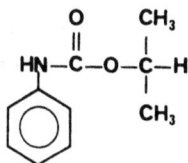

$$C_{10}H_{13}NO_2 \qquad \text{Mol. wt: } 179.2$$

1.3 Chemical and physical properties of the substance

From Weast (1975), unless otherwise specified

(a) Description: White needles

(b) Melting-point: $90^{\circ}C$

(c) Refractive index: n_D^{91} 1.4989

(d) Spectroscopy data: λ_{max} 236 nm and 274 nm (E_1^1 = 46 and 942); for infra-red spectra, see Grasselli (1973)

(e) Solubility: Insoluble in water at room temperature; soluble in most organic solvents (Stecher, 1968)

1.4 Technical products and impurities

Propham is available in the US as an emulsifiable concentrate containing about 24% of the active ingredient, in granule forms containing 10% and 15%, as a flowable suspension containing about 48% and as a wettable powder containing 50% of the chemical (Berg, 1975).

2. Production, Use, Occurrence and Analysis

For important background information on this section, see preamble, p. 15.

2.1 Production and use

Propham can be prepared either by the reaction of phenyl isocyanate with isopropyl alcohol or by the reaction of isopropyl chloroformate with aniline.

Propham was first produced commercially in the US in 1946 (US Tariff Commission, 1947; only one company now produces it there (US Tariff Commission, 1968). There have been no imports into the US since 1971, when 2500 kg were imported. Propham is reported to be produced in The Netherlands and the UK (Berg, 1975) but not in Japan.

Its plant-growth regulatory properties were first reported in 1945 (Spencer, 1973), and it is used as a selective pre-planting, pre-emergence and post-emergence herbicide. It effectively controls many annual grassy weeds and certain broadleaf weeds and is registered in the US for use on about 12 forage, field and vegetable crops at residue tolerances ranging from 0.1 to 5 mg/kg (US Environmental Protection Agency, 1974).

About 200 thousand kg propham were used on agricultural crops in the US in 1971. More than half of the 60 thousand kg used in the state of California in 1974 was applied to sugar beets; a total of 30 thousand acres of cropland were so treated (California Department of Food & Agriculture, 1975).

It was determined from a questionnaire sent to a number of herbicide manufacturers that a 'small' amount of propham is used in Italy as a potato sprout inhibitor.

190

2.2 Occurrence

Propham is not known to occur as a natural product. Residual amounts
may be present on or in treated crops after harvesting.

2.3 Analysis

Several reviews include methods of analysis for propham (Fishbein &
Zielinski, 1967; Gard & Ferguson, 1964; Zweig & Sherma, 1972). Various
methods of analysis suitable for propham are described in the monograph
on chloropropham (Burge & Gross, 1972; Frei & Lawrence, 1973; Lawrence
& Laver, 1974, 1975). A thin-layer chromatographic method for the
identification of sixty-one pesticides, including propham, is reported
by Ebing (1972).

Colorimetric measurement of the alkaline distillation product may
be adapted to the analysis of propham residues in a wide range of fruits
and vegetables (Ferguson & Gard, 1969).

3. Biological Data Relevant to the Evaluation
of Carcinogenic Risk to Man

3.1 Carcinogenicity and related studies in animals

(a) Oral administration

Mouse: A group of 50 12-week old mice (strain and sex unspecified)
was fed 0.1% propham (purity unspecified) in the diet for 18 months, when
the survivors were killed. The treatment produced signs of toxicity, and
the animals were returned to the normal diet at intervals. Fifteen mice
were dead by 6 months, and only 2 survived 12-18 months. No tumours were
observed. A further group of 50 'C' mice (25 of each sex) was fed 0.5%
propham in the diet for 18 months, when the survivors were killed. The
treatment produced signs of toxicity, and the animals were returned to the
normal diet at intervals. Twenty mice were dead by 6 months, and 16
survived 12-18 months. No tumours were observed (Hueper, 1952).

Groups of 18 male and 18 female (C57BL/6xC3H/Anf)F_1 mice and 18 male
and 18 female (C57BL/6xAKR)F_1 mice received propham (100% pure) according to
the following schedule: 215 mg/kg bw in gelatine at 7 days of age by

191

stomach tube and the same amount (not adjusted for increasing body weight) daily up to 4 weeks of age; subsequently, the mice were given 560 mg propham per kg of diet. The dose was the maximum tolerated dose for infant and young mice but not necessarily so for adults. The experiment was terminated when the mice were about 78 weeks of age, at which time 11, 17, 14 and 16 mice in the four groups, respectively, were still alive. Tumour incidences were compared with those observed among 79-90 necropsied mice of each sex and strain, which either had been untreated or had received gelatine only: the incidences were not significantly increased (P>0.05) for any tumour type in any sex-strain subgroup or in the combined sexes of either strain (Innes *et al.*, 1969; NTIS, 1968).

Rat: Fifteen 32-week old Osborne-Mendel rats (sex unspecified) were fed 2% propham (purity unspecified) (20 g/kg of diet), alternating with 1-2 weeks of normal diet, for 18 months, when the 8 survivors were killed. No tumours were found; however, histological examination of only 6 rats was carried out (Hueper, 1952).

Two groups of 9 white rats each received 10 mg propham (m.p. 87°C) as a 3% oily solution daily in the diet for 18 months, or 15 mg as a 5% mixture with kaolin powder in the diet for 15 months. Six rats of the second group and 3 of the first were killed before 8 months; no lung tumours were found (Engelhorn, 1954).

Hamster: A group of 23 male and 26 female 6-week old golden hamsters were fed 2 g propham (m.p. about 87°C) per kg of diet for 33 months and were compared with an untreated group of 22 males and 27 females. After 2 years, 6 treated and 1 control female and 13 treated and 14 control males were still alive. Bile-duct hyperplasia of the liver was observed in 28 treated animals and in 28 controls. A total of 6 tumours in different organs was seen in treated animals, compared with 8 in controls (van Esch & Kroes, 1972).

(b) Subcutaneous and/or intramuscular administration

Mouse: Of 35 female and 39 male 20-week old C mice injected in the right femoral muscle with 400 mg/kg bw propham (purity unspecified) in 0.1 ml lanolin every second week for 6 months and observed for a further year, only 15 females and 3 males survived 13 or more months; no tumours were observed (Hueper, 1952).

Groups of 18 male and 18 female (C57BL/6xC3H/Anf)F$_1$ mice and 18 male and 18 female (C57BL/6xAKR)F$_1$ mice were given single s.c. injections of 215 mg/kg bw propham (100% pure) in dimethyl sulphoxide on the 28th day of life and were observed until they were about 78 weeks of age, at which time 16, 18, 17 and 17 mice in the four groups, respectively, were still alive. Tumour incidences were compared with those in groups of 141, 154, 161 and 157 untreated or vehicle-injected controls that were necropsied. Incidences were not increased (P>0.05) for any tumour type in any sex-strain subgroup or in combined sexes of either strain (NTIS, 1968) [The Working Group noted that a negative result obtained with a single s.c. injection may not be an adequate basis for discounting carcinogenicity].

Rat: Fifteen 24-week old female Osborne-Mendel rats were injected in the right femoral muscle with 400 mg/kg bw propham (purity unspecified) in 0.2 ml lanolin once a month for 6 months and were observed for a further year. Three rats died before the 13th month of the experiment. Tumours found in 4/10 necropsied rats were 1 adenofibroma in the region of the groin, 2 adenomyomas of the uterus and 1 adenocarcinoma of the breast. One mammary adenoma was found among 10 control rats (Hueper, 1952).

(c) Intraperitoneal injection

Mouse: A group of 16 7-9-week old male A/He mice was given 12 i.p. injections of 5 mg/animal propham (purity unspecified) in tricaprylin over a period of 4 weeks and killed 20 weeks after the end of treatment. Only the incidence of lung tumours is reported: 1 was found in 1/10 survivors, compared with 8 in 7/28 controls receiving the solvent only and 2 in 2/31 untreated mice; with a dose of only 3.2 mg, 2/14 surviving mice developed lung tumours (Shimkin et al., 1969).

(d) Other experimental systems

Intrapleural injection: A group of 30 male and 30 female C mice was given repeated intrapleural injections of 400 mg/kg bw propham (purity unspecified) in 0.1 ml lanolin every second week for 6 months. Only 9 females survived more than 13 months. No tumours were observed, although 2 females had 'white nodular masses in the lungs' (Hueper, 1952).

A group of 15 20-week old male rats was given repeated intrapleural injections of 400 mg/kg bw propham (purity unspecified) in 0.2 ml lanolin monthly for 6 months. Only 9 rats were autopsied; 6 of these lived for less than 14 months. No tumours were found (Hueper, 1952).

Oral administration with skin application of a promoting agent: Groups of 15 Swiss mice of each sex received propham (m.p. 84°C) according to one of the following schedules: (1) a single dose of 15 mg/animal as a 1% solution in tragacanth given by stomach tube; (2) 15 mg once weekly for 10 weeks; or (3) 1 g/kg of diet (0.1%) for 6 months. Promotion was induced either with a 5% solution of croton oil in olive oil twice weekly or with undiluted Tween 60 given 6 times/week for 6 months. Six months after the start of the experiment, the proportions of mice (males and females considered together) with skin papillomas were as follows:

Propham	Croton oil		Tween 60	
	Papilloma-bearing animals	Papillomas per animal	Papilloma-bearing animals	Papillomas per animal
15 mg x 1	4/27	1.3	0/26	0.0
15 mg x 10	8/28	1.3	1/25	3.0
1 g/kg of diet	6/27	5.2	1/25	2.0
None	1/22	1.0	1/27	2.0

Animals with papillomas were observed for a further 10 months. A total of 65 papillomas appeared during the 6 months of treatment plus 10 months of observation in mice given propham and croton oil; 4 of these were still present 6 months after the end of treatment, and in 2 animals the papillomas progressed to carcinomas. Only 1 papilloma was seen in controls receiving croton oil only. In mice given propham and Tween 60, 5 papillomas appeared during the two periods. No skin tumours occurred in similar groups of mice given the propham treatments without the croton oil or Tween 60 treatments (van Esch et al., 1958).

In a further experiment, a group of 50 Swiss <u>mice</u> of each sex received 15 mg/animal propham by stomach tube 10 times weekly and then twice weekly cutaneous applications of croton oil for 26 weeks. It is reported that "a clear increase was observed in the number of males with papillomas, and in both sexes, in the total number of papillomas. In the males, two malignant tumours were present" (van Esch *et al.*, 1965, reported in van Esch & Kroes, 1972).

3.2 Other relevant biological data

(a) Experimental systems

In rats, the oral LD_{50} of propham is 1-9 g/kg bw (Ben-Dyke *et al.*, 1970). Groups of mice were given 1-20 g propham per kg of diet for about 18 months. At levels of 1 and 5 g/kg of diet, animals became emaciated, and some died unless they were transferred from the propham-containing diet every 2 weeks and fed the normal diet for a similar period; mortality was high in animals fed 10 and 20 g/kg of diet. Fifteen rats survived administration of 20 g propham per kg of diet for 18 months when they were given alternately the propham-containing diet for 1-2 months and a normal diet for 1-2 weeks (Hueper, 1952).

After oral administration of [isopropyl-^{14}C]- and [ring-^{14}C]-labelled propham to rats, the 3-day urinary excretions of herbicide-related material represented 80 and 85% of the dose, respectively; in the case of the isopropyl-labelled compound, an additional 5% of the dose was excreted as carbon dioxide *via* the lungs. There was no significant difference in the rate of excretion or eliminative route among rats receiving oral doses ranging from 4-200 mg/kg bw. Herbicide-related material was distributed thoughout the body, with highest concentrations in the kidneys. A small degree of herbicide hydrolysis occurred in neomycin-treated rats, probably in the liver. Approximately 30% of an i.v. dose of propham was excreted in the 6-hour bile (Bend *et al.*, 1971; Fang *et al.*, 1974).

In a lactating goat given a single dose of 100 mg/kg bw propham (1) (Scheme 1), the urinary metabolites included conjugates of isopropyl 4-hydroxycarbanilate (2), isopropyl 3,4-dihydroxycarbanilate (3), isopropyl 2-hydroxycarbanilate (4), (2-hydroxyisopropyl)-4-hydroxycarbanilate (5),

SCHEME 1

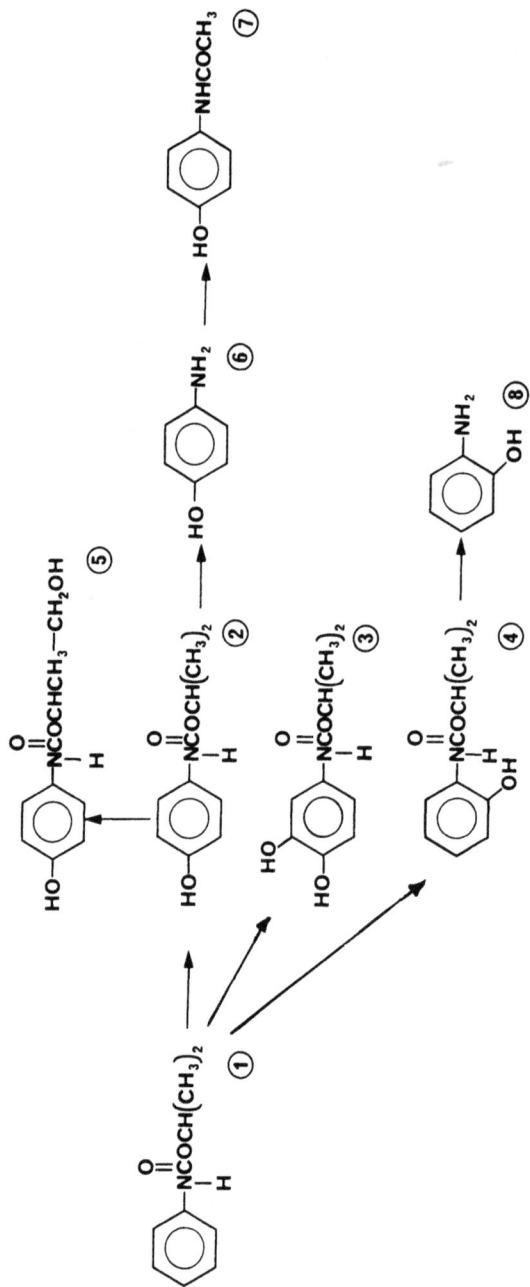

4-hydroxyaniline (6), 4-hydroxyacetanilide (7) and 2-hydroxyaniline (8).
Small amounts of propham metabolites were also excreted in the faeces and
milk (Paulson *et al.*, 1973). Similarly, in the urine of rats treated with
propham (1) 80% of the dose occurred as the sulphate ester of isopropyl
4-hydroxycarbanilate (2) together with other conjugates (Bend *et al.*, 1971;
Fang *et al.*, 1974; Holder & Ryan, 1968; Paulson *et al.*, 1973).

Propham inhibits spindle fibre formation and induces chromosome
aberrations in plants (Amer & Farah, 1974; Coss *et al.*, 1975). No reverse
mutations were detected in *Bacillus subtilis* (De Giovanni-Donnelly *et al.*,
1968) or in *Salmonella typhimurium* (Andersen *et al.*, 1972); metabolic
activation systems were not used in the tests on bacteria.

(b) Man

No data were available to the Working Group.

3.3 Case reports and epidemiological studies

No data were available to the Working Group.

4. Comments on Data Reported and Evaluation

4.1 Animal data

In one study in which propham was administered orally to two strains
of mice, no evidence of carcinogenicity was observed. Other studies in mice,
rats and hamsters by oral administration, in mice and rats by subcutaneous
injection and in mice by intraperitoneal or intrapleural injection also
showed no carcinogenicity, but they were inadequate either in terms of
the number of surviving animals, the total dose or the extent of pathology
carried out. Orally administered propham acted as an initiator in two-stage
carcinogenesis studies in mice.

4.2 Human data

No case reports or epidemiological studies were available to the
Working Group.

5. References

Amer, S.M. & Farah, O.R. (1974) Cytological effects of pesticides. VII. Mitotic effects of isopropyl-*N*-phenyl carbamate and 'Duphar'. Cytologia, 40, 21-29

Andersen, K.J., Leighty, E.G. & Takahashi, M.T. (1972) Evaluation of herbicides for possible mutagenic properties. J. agric. Fd Chem., 20, 649-656

Bend, J.R., Holder, G.M. & Ryan, A.J. (1971) Further studies on the metabolism of isopropyl *N*-phenylcarbamate (propham) in the rat. Fd Cosmet. Toxicol., 9, 169-177

Ben-Dyke, R., Sanderson, D.M. & Noakes, D.N. (1970) Acute toxicity data for pesticides. Wld Rev. Pest. Control, 9, 119-127

Berg, G.L., ed. (1975) Farm Chemicals Handbook 1975, Willoughby, Ohio, Meister, p. D 113

Burge, W.D. & Gross, L.E. (1972) Determination of IPC, CIPC and propanil and some metabolites of these herbicides in soil incubation studies. Soil Sci., 114, 440-443

California Department of Food and Agriculture (1975) Pesticide Use Report, 1974, Sacramento, p. 86

Coss, R.A., Bloodgood, R.A., Brower, D.L., Pickett-Heaps, J.D. & McIntosh, J.R. (1975) Studies on the mechanism of action of isopropyl *N*-phenyl carbamate. Exp. Cell Res., 92, 394-398

De Giovanni-Donnelly, R., Kolbye, S.M. & Greeves, P.D. (1968) Effect of IPC, CIPC, sevin and zectran on *Bacillus subtilis*. Experientia, 24, 80-81

Ebing, W. (1972) Routinemethode zur dünnschichtchromatographischen Identifizierung der Pestizidrückstände aus den Klassen der Triazine, Carbamate, Harnstoffe und Uracile. J. Chromat., 65, 533-545

Engelhorn, R. (1954) Über den Einfluss des Äthyl-Urethans und des Phenylcarbaminsäure-isopropylesters auf das Lungengewebe der Ratte. Arch. exp. Path. Pharmakol., 223, 177-181

van Esch, G.J. & Kroes, R. (1972) Long-term toxicity studies of chloropropham and propham in mice and hamsters. Fd Cosmet. Toxicol., 10, 373-381

van Esch, G.J., van Genderen, H. & Vink, H.H. (1958) The production of skin tumours in mice by oral treatment with urethane, isopropyl-*N*-phenylcarbamate or isopropyl-*N*-chlorophenylcarbamate in combination with skin painting with croton oil and Tween 60. Brit. J. Cancer, 12, 355-362

Fang, S.C., Fallin, E., Montgomery, M.L. & Freed, V.H. (1974) Metabolic studies of ^{14}C-labelled propham and chlorpropham in the female rat. Pest. Biochem. Physiol., 4, 1-11

Ferguson, C.E. & Gard, L. (1969) IPC and CIPC residue analysis. J. agric. Fd Chem., 17, 1062-1065

Fishbein, L. & Zielinski, W.L., Jr (1967) Chromatography of carbamates. Chromat. Rev., 9, 37-101

Frei, R.W. & Lawrence, J.F. (1973) Fluorigenic labelling in high-speed liquid chromatography. J. Chromat., 83, 321-330

Gard, L.N. & Ferguson, C.E., Jr (1964) IPC. In: Zweig, G., ed., Analytical Methods for Pesticides, Plant Growth Regulators and Food Additives, Vol. 4, Herbicides, New York, Academic Press, pp. 139-145

Grasselli, J.G., ed. (1973) Atlas of Spectral Data and Physical Constants for Organic Components, Cleveland, Ohio, Chemical Rubber Co., p. B-400

Holder, G.M. & Ryan, A.J. (1968) Metabolism of propham (isopropyl N-phenyl-carbamate) in the rat. Nature (Lond.), 220, 77

Hueper, W.C. (1952) Carcinogenic studies on isopropyl-N-phenyl-carbamate. Industr. Med. Surg., 21, 71-74

Innes, J.R.M., Ulland, B.M., Valerio, M.G., Petrucelli, L., Fishbein, L., Hart, E.R., Pallotta, A.J., Bates, R.R., Falk, H.L., Gart, J.J., Klein, M., Mitchell, I. & Peters, J. (1969) Bioassay of pesticides and industrial chemicals for tumorigenicity in mice: a preliminary note. J. nat. Cancer Inst., 42, 1101-1114

Lawrence, J.F. & Laver, G.W. (1974) Analysis of carbamate and urea herbicides in foods, using fluorogenic labeling. J. Ass. off. analyt. Chem., 57, 1022-1025

Lawrence, J.F. & Laver, G.W. (1975) Analysis of some carbamate and urea herbicides in foods by gas-liquid chromatography after alkylation. J. agric. Fd Chem., 23, 1106-1109

NTIS (National Technical Information Service) (1968) Evaluation of Carcino-genic, Teratogenic and Mutagenic Activities of Selected Pesticides and Industrial Chemicals, Vol. 1, Carcinogenic Study, Washington DC, US Department of Commerce

Paulson, G.D., Jacobsen, A.M., Zaylskie, R.G. & Feil, V.J. (1973) Isolation and identification of propham (isopropyl carbanilate) metabolites from the rat and goat. J. agric. Fd Chem., 21, 804-811

Shimkin, M.B., Wieder, R., McDonough, M., Fishbein, L. & Swern, D. (1969) Lung tumor response in strain A mice as a quantitative bioassay of carcinogenic activity of some carbamates and aziridines. Cancer Res., 29, 2184-2190

Spencer, E.Y. (1973) Guide to the Chemicals Used in Crop Protection, 6th ed., London, Ontario, University of Western Ontario, Research Branch, Agriculture Canada, Publication 1093, p. 431

Stecher, P.G., ed. (1968) The Merck Index, 8th ed., Rahway, NJ, Merck & Co., p. 575

US Environmental Protection Agency (1974) EPA Compendium of Registered Pesticides, Washington DC, US Government Printing office, pp. I-I-5.1-I-I-5.3

US Tariff Commission (1947) Synthetic Organic Chemicals, US Production and Sales, 1946, Report No. 159, Second Series, Washington DC, US Government Printing Office, p. 135

US Tariff Commission (1968) Synthetic Organic Chemicals, US Production and Sales, 1966, TC Publication 248, Washington DC, US Government Printing Office, p. 178

Weast, R.C., ed. (1975) CRC Handbook of Chemistry and Physics, 56th ed., Cleveland, Ohio, Chemical Rubber Co., p. C-232

Zweig, G. & Sherma, J. (1972) IPC. In: Zweig, G., ed., Analytical Methods for Pesticides, Plant Growth Regulators and Food Additives, Vol. 6, Gas Chromatographic Analysis, New York, Academic Press, pp. 657-658

n-PROPYL CARBAMATE

1. Chemical and Physical Data

1.1 Synonyms and trade names

Chem. Abstr. Reg. Serial No.: 627-12-3

Chem. Abstr. Name: Carbamic acid, propyl ester

Propyl carbamate; propyl urethane

1.2 Chemical formula and molecular weight

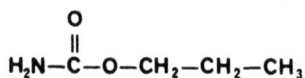

$$H_2N-\overset{\overset{\textstyle O}{\|}}{C}-O-CH_2-CH_2-CH_3$$

$$C_4H_9NO_2 \qquad \text{Mol. wt: } 103.1$$

1.3 Chemical and physical properties of the substance

From Weast (1975), unless otherwise specified

(a) Description: Prisms

(b) Boiling-point: $196^{\circ}C$; $92-92.5^{\circ}C$ at 12 mm

(c) Melting-point: $60^{\circ}C$

(d) Spectroscopy data: For infra-red spectral data, see Grasselli (1973)

(e) Solubility: Soluble in water, ethanol and diethyl ether (Prager & Jacobson, 1921)

(f) Volatility: Vapour pressure is 1 mm at $52.4^{\circ}C$ (Jordan, 1954).

1.4 Technical products and impurities

No data were available to the Working Group.

2. Production, Use, Occurrence and Analysis

For important background information on this section, see preamble, p. 15.

2.1 Production and use

n-Propyl carbamate was first synthesized by heating urea with excess propyl alcohol by Cahours in 1873 (Prager & Jacobson, 1921). It can be prepared by treating n-propyl alcohol with cyanogen chloride in the presence of hydrochloric acid (Fuks & Hartemink, 1973).

Commercial production of n-propyl carbamate was first reported in the US in 1966 (US Tariff Commission, 1968). Production by one manufacturer in 1972 was estimated to be 45 thousand kg; one manufacturer reported production in 1973 (US International Trade Commission, 1975).

Propyl carbamate (isomer unspecified) is believed to be used as a chemical intermediate in the manufacture of dimethylol propyl carbamate-based resins which are used in the textile industry as durable-press fabric finishes for cotton and polyester/cotton blends. Textiles treated with these resins have improved durability and wash-and-wear properties (Ramunda *et al.*, 1973).

2.2 Occurrence

n-Propyl carbamate is not known to occur as a natural product.

2.3 Analysis

Methods for the chromatographic analysis of carbamates, including alkyl carbamates, have been reviewed (Fishbein & Zielinski, 1967). A gas chromatographic method has been described for detection of microgram amounts of n-propyl carbamate in a mixture of alkyl carbamates after the formation of their trimethylsilyl derivatives (Nery, 1969).

A thin-layer chromatographic method for the separation of short-chain alkyl carbamates on silica gel with a complex solvent system has been reported (Knappe & Rohdewald, 1966). The separated materials from this procedure are identified by hydrolysis and conversion to the 3,5-dinitro-benzoate derivative (Valk & Schliefer, 1967).

202

3. Biological Data Relevant to the Evaluation of Carcinogenic Risk to Man

3.1 Carcinogenicity and related studies in animals

(a) Intraperitoneal administration

Mouse: A group of 32 10-12-week old strain A mice (approximately equally divided by sex) were given 13 weekly i.p. injections of 0.5 mg/mouse commercial n-propyl carbamate (purity unspecified) and were killed 2 weeks after the end of the treatment, when they were 6 months old: 19 developed lung tumours, with an average of 0.9 tumours/mouse. An additional group of 46 mice received the same treatment with recrystallized n-propyl carbamate; lung tumours developed in 30 animals, with an average of 1.0 lung tumour/mouse. Lung tumours were found in 24/141 untreated controls, with a mean of 0.18 tumours/mouse (Larsen, 1947) [P<0.001].

A group of 52 6-8-week old C57BL6 mice (approximately equally divided by sex) received 10 weekly i.p. injections of 570 mg/kg bw n-propyl carbamate (purity unspecified) and were autopsied 62 weeks after the start of treatment. One mouse died with leukaemia at 17 weeks; 7/44 mice which survived to the end of the experiment developed lung adenomas (P>0.05), with an average of 0.2 tumours/mouse. Of another group, which had been exposed also to total body irradiation with 400R 1 week before the chemical was administered, 3/50 mice died with leukaemia within 38 weeks. Of untreated controls, 9/75 developed lung adenomas; the incidence of leukaemia in this strain was reported to be 0.7% (Mirvish et al., 1969).

A group of 17 6-8-week old Swiss mice (approximately equally divided by sex) received 5 weekly i.p. injections of 570 mg/kg bw n-propyl carbamate (purity 80-100%) in water and were killed 14 months after the start of the experiment. In another group of 38 mice, this treatment was followed one week later by twice weekly skin applications of 5% croton oil in liquid paraffin for 40 weeks; the survivors were killed 14 months after the start of the experiment. No skin tumours were found in either group. Two mice treated with n-propyl carbamate plus croton oil died with leukaemia, compared with 0/50 controls given croton oil only. At the end of the experiment, 16 of a total of 21 survivors that had received n-propyl carbamate (with or without subsequent croton oil treatment) had lung adenomas (average, 1.5 tumours per mouse). The incidence of lung adenomas in controls given croton oil only was 3/17, with an average of 0.4 tumours/mouse (Mirvish *et al.*, 1969).

A group of 16 7-9-week old male A/He mice were given 12 i.p. injections of 5 mg *n*-propyl carbamate in tricaprylin over a period of 4 weeks and were killed 20 weeks after the end of treatment. Only incidences of lung tumours were reported: lung adenomas (1 adenoma/animal) were found in 9/12 mice given *n*-propyl carbamate, in 7/28 mice given the solvent only (one mouse with 2 tumours) and in 2/31 untreated controls (Shimkin *et al.*, 1969).

(b) Other experimental systems

Oral administration and skin promotion: A group of 20 8-12-week old Swiss mice received a single oral administration of 25 mg *n*-propyl carbamate in water, followed 4 days later by twice-weekly applications of a 5% solution of croton oil in liquid paraffin on the dorsal skin for 40 weeks. Within 20 weeks, 3/15 survivors developed skin tumours (average, 0.2 tumours/mouse), compared with 3/45 (0.07 tumours/mouse) in controls treated with croton oil only. By the end of the treatment, 4/14 animals had developed skin tumours (0.3 skin tumours/mouse), compared with 11/44 (0.4 skin tumours/mouse) in the croton oil-treated control group. Lung adenomas were found in 4/14 animals of the experimental group and in 2/42 of the croton oil-treated controls (Berenblum *et al.*, 1959).

Subcutaneous injection and skin promotion: A group of 40 7-week old male 'Hall' mice were given single s.c. injections of 20 mg *n*-propyl carbamate in saline. Treatment was followed 2 weeks later by 24 weekly cutaneous applications within 26 weeks of 0.25 ml of a 0.07% solution of croton oil in acetone. Of 26 mice injected with *n*-propyl carbamate and still alive 1 week after the end of the croton oil treatment, 5 developed skin tumours (1 tumour/mouse). Of controls receiving croton oil only, 2/41 developed a total of 3 skin tumours. No tumours occurred in mice that received a single injection of *n*-propyl carbamate and were observed for 26 weeks (Pound, 1967) [P>0.05].

Injection and skin promotion: Two groups of 29 and 27 7-week old male 'Hall' mice were given a single injection (route unspecified) of 7.7 mEq/kg bw *n*-propyl carbamate. Eighteen hours before this treatment, the second group received an application of 0.24 ml of a 0.075% croton oil solution in acetone over the whole area of the dorsal skin. Three weeks later, both groups were given 32 weekly treatments with croton oil, each application consisting of 0.24 ml of a 0.075% solution in acetone during the first 18 weeks and 0.15% for a further 14 weeks. A control group of 90 mice received croton oil only. The numbers of mice with skin tumours still alive at 36 weeks were 3/24 in the group which had had no preliminary croton oil treatment, 3/27 in the second group and 8/86 in controls. The numbers of skin tumours, hepatomas, liver haemangiomas, lung adenomas or leukaemias were not statistically increased in mice that survived up to 78 weeks, in comparison to controls (Pound & Lawson, 1976).

3.2 Other relevant biological data

(a) Experimental systems

The s.c. LD_{50} of *n*-propyl carbamate in mice is 1.3 g/kg bw (Pound, 1967).

Rats injected intraperitoneally with *n*-propyl carbamate or the corresponding *N*-hydroxycarbamate excrete both the carbamate and *N*-hydroxycarbamate in the urine (Boyland & Nery, 1965). The binding of [^{14}C-propyl]-*n*-propyl carbamate to the DNA of mouse liver was very low compared with that of [^{14}C-ethyl]-ethyl carbamate (Lawson & Pound, 1973).

Pregnant Syrian hamsters were injected intraperitoneally on day 8 of gestation with *n*-propyl carbamate or one of a series of structurally-related carbamates. In foetuses examined on day 13 of gestation, the effects of *n*-propyl carbamate were compared with those of urethane; it was found (i) to have been as teratogenic, (ii) to have given the same kind of malformations and (iii) to have retarded growth to the same extent. The numbers of dead foetuses and resorptions that were produced by treatment with propyl and ethyl carbamates were similar (DiPaolo & Elis, 1967).

No reverse mutations were induced in *Bacillus subtilis* (De Giovanni-Donnelly *et al.*, 1967); metabolic activation systems were not used in this test.

(b) Man

No data were available to the Working Group.

3.3 Case reports and epidemiological studies

No data were available to the Working Group.

4. Comments on Data Reported and Evaluation[1]

4.1 Animal data

n-Propyl carbamate is carcinogenic in mice after its intraperitoneal injection: it produced lung adenomas in three different strains [For a comparison with ethyl carbamate (urethane), see IARC (1974)].

4.2 Human data

No case reports or epidemiological studies were available to the Working Group.

_____

[1]See also the section, 'Animal data in relation to the evaluation of risk to man' in the introduction to this volume, p. 13.

5. References

Berenblum, I., Ben-Ishai, D., Haran-Ghera, N., Lapidot, A., Simon, E. &
Trainin, N. (1959) Skin initiating action and lung carcinogenesis by
derivatives of urethane (ethyl carbamate) and related compounds.
Biochem. Pharmacol., 2, 168-176

Boyland, E. & Nery, R. (1965) The metabolism of urethane and related
compounds. Biochem. J., 94, 198-208

De Giovanni-Donnelly, R., Kolbye, S.M. & DiPaolo, J.A. (1967) Effect of
carbamates on *Bacillus subtilis*. Mutation Res., 4, 543-551

DiPaolo, J.A. & Elis, J. (1967) The comparison of teratogenic and carcinogenic effects of some carbamate compounds. Cancer Res., 27, 1696-1701

Fishbein, L. & Zielinski, W.L., Jr (1967) Chromatography of carbamates.
Chromat. Rev., 9, 37-101

Fuks, R. & Hartemink, M.A. (1973) Acid-catalysed reaction of cyanogen
chloride with aliphatic alcohols. General synthesis of aliphatic
carbamates. Bull. Soc. chim. belg., 82, 23-30

Grasselli, J.G., ed. (1973) Atlas of Spectral Data and Physical Constants
for Organic Compounds, Cleveland, Ohio, Chemical Rubber Co., p. B-398

IARC (1974) IARC Monographs on the Evaluation of Carcinogenic Risk of
Chemicals to Man, 7, Some Anti-thyroid and Related Substances,
Nitrofurans and Industrial Chemicals, Lyon, pp. 111-140

Jordan, T.E. (1954) Vapor Pressure of Organic Compounds, New York,
Interscience, pp. 179, 192

Knappe, E. & Rohdewald, I. (1966) Dünnschichtchromatographie von substituierten Harnstoffen und einfachen Urethanen. Z. analyt. Chem., 217, 110-113

Larsen, C.D. (1947) Evaluation of the carcinogenicity of a series of
esters of carbamic acid. J. nat. Cancer Inst., 8, 99-101

Lawson, T.A. & Pound, A.W. (1973) The interaction of carbon-14-labelled
alkyl carbamates, labelled in the alkyl and carbonyl positions, with
DNA *in vivo*. Chem.-biol. Interact., 6, 99-105

Mirvish, S.S., Chen, L., Haran-Ghera, N. & Berenblum, I. (1969) Comparative
study of lung carcinogenesis, promoting action in leukaemogenesis and
initiating action in skin tumorigenesis by urethane, hydrazine and
related compounds. Int. J. Cancer, 4, 318-326

Nery, R. (1969) Gas-chromatographic determination of acetyl and trimethyl-silyl derivatives of alkyl carbamates and their *N*-hydroxy derivatives. Analyst, 94, 130-135

Pound, A.W. (1967) The initiation of skin tumours in mice by homologues and *N*-substituted derivatives of ethyl carbamate. Austr. J. exp. Biol. med. Sci., 45, 507-516

Pound, A.W. & Lawson, T.A. (1976) Carcinogenesis by carbamic acid esters and their binding to DNA. Cancer Res., 36, 1101-1107

Prager, B. & Jacobson, P., eds (1921) Beilsteins Handbuch der organischen Chemie, 4th ed., Vol. 3, Syst. No. 201, pp. 28-29

Ramunda, A.J., Adams, P., Beinfest, S. & Gulakowski, T.A. (1973) Treatment of cellulosic fiber-containing fabrics to improve their physical characteristics. US Patent 3,752,697, August 14, to Millmaster Onyx Corp.

Shimkin, M.B., Wieder, R., McDonough, M., Fishbein, L. & Swern, D. (1969) Lung tumor response in strain A mice as a quantitative bioassay of carcinogenic activity of some carbamates and aziridines. Cancer Res., 29, 2184-2190

US International Trade Commission (1975) Synthetic Organic Chemicals, US Production and Sales, 1973, ITC Publication 728, Washington DC, US Government Printing Office, p. 218

US Tariff Commission (1968) Synthetic Organic Chemicals, US Production and Sales, 1966, TC Publication 248, Washington DC, US Government Printing Office, p. 178

Valk, G. & Schliefer, K. (1967) Trennung und Nachweis von cyclischen Harnstoff-Derivaten und Carbamaten sowie deren Hydrolyseprodukten durch Dünnschicht-chromatographie. Textilindustrie, 69, 783-786

Weast, R.C., ed. (1975) CRC Handbook of Chemistry and Physics, 56th ed., Cleveland, Ohio, Chemical Rubber Co., p. C-231

SEMICARBAZIDE (HYDROCHLORIDE)

1. Chemical and Physical Data

1.1 Synonyms and trade names

Chem. Abstr. Reg. Serial No.: 563-41-7

Chem. Abstr. Name: Hydrazinecarboxamide monohydrochloride

Amidourea hydrochloride; aminourea hydrochloride; carbamylhydrazine hydrochloride; semicarbazide monohydrochloride

1.2 Chemical formula and molecular weight

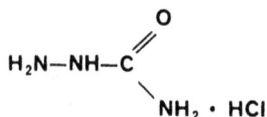

$$H_2N-NH-C \overset{\displaystyle O}{\underset{\displaystyle NH_2 \cdot HCl}{\Big\langle}}$$

CH_6ClN_3O Mol. wt: 111.5

1.3 Chemical and physical properties of the substance

From Weast (1975), unless otherwise specified

(a) Description: Prisms

(b) Melting-point: 175-177°C (with decomposition)

(c) Spectroscopy data: λ_{max} = 278 nm and 357 nm (E_1^1 = 0.5 and 1.1) in water; for infra-red spectral data, see Grasselli (1973)

(d) Solubility: Soluble in water; very slightly soluble in hot ethanol; insoluble in anhydrous ether (Stecher, 1968)

1.4 Technical products and impurities

Semicarbazide hydrochloride is available commercially in the US in chemically pure and technical grades (Hawley, 1971).

2. Production, Use, Occurrence and Analysis

For important background information on this section, see preamble, p. 15.

2.1 Production and use

The first reported preparation of semicarbazide hydrochloride was by reaction of benzylidenesemicarbazide with hydrochloric acid (Thiele & Stange, 1894). It can also be produced by the electrochemical reduction of nitrourea in aqueous hydrochloric acid (Korczynski, 1969). The method used for commercial production is not known.

Commercial production of semicarbazide hydrochloride was first reported in the US in 1940 (US Tariff Commission, 1941); in 1974, one manufacturer reported production (US International Trade Commission, 1975). It is produced in the UK for research purposes.

Semicarbazide hydrochloride has been used as a chemical reagent in the qualitative determination of aldehydes and ketones (Stecher, 1968) and in the isolation of hormones and of certain fractions from essential oils (Hawley, 1971).

2.2 Occurrence

Semicarbazide hydrochloride is not known to occur as a natural product.

2.3 Analysis

A potentiometric method for the measurement of semicarbazide hydrochloride, sensitive to at least 0.3 mg, has been described (Pszonicka & Skwara, 1970).

3. Biological Data Relevant to the Evaluation of Carcinogenic Risk to Man[1]

3.1 Carcinogenicity and related studies in animals

(a) Oral administration

Mouse: An unspecified number of 6-8-week old female dd mice were fed a diet containing 0.1% semicarbazide hydrochloride for 7 months. At the end of treatment, 8 survivors were killed and examined for lung tumours: 6 mice had a total of 8 lung tumours, compared with 1 tumour in 20 controls (Mori et al., 1960) [P<0.001].

Commercial semicarbazide hydrochloride was administered to 25 male and 25 female 6-week old Swiss mice for lifetime as a 0.0625% solution in the drinking-water. The average daily intakes were 3.3 mg/female and 4.8 mg/male; lifespan was reduced in treated males. In females, 37 lung tumours occurred in 25/50 treated animals (0.7 tumours/mouse), compared with 31 in 21/99 female controls (0.3 tumours/mouse) [P<0.001]; there was no increase in the incidence of lung tumours in treated males. Tumours of vascular origin were observed at various sites in 9/50 treated females, compared with 5/99 female controls [P<0.02], and in 3/50 treated males (4 tumours), compared with 6/99 male controls [P>0.05]. The 13 blood-vessel tumours in treated mice included 6 angiosarcomas and 2 angiomas of the liver. Other tumours were equally distributed among treated and control mice (Toth & Shimizu, 1974; Toth et al., 1975).

Rat: A 2-year feeding study with semicarbazide in Charles River CD rats has been described (Ulland et al., 1973) [The inadequate reporting does not allow an evaluation of this experiment].

---

[1]Semicarbazide is a hydrazine derivative. For a discussion of hydrazine and related substances, see IARC (1974).

3.2 Other relevant biological data

(a) Experimental systems

The s.c., i.p., i.v. and oral LD_{50} doses for semicarbazide in mice range from 123-176 mg/kg bw. The compound is a convulsant (Jenney & Pfeiffer, 1958).

The offspring of pregnant rats treated orally with semicarbazide during pregnancy had facial abnormalities, including micrognathia and cleft palates (Stivers *et al.*, 1971).

Administration of 50 or 100 mg/day to pregnant Sprague-Dawley rats on days 10-16 of gestation produced a high incidence of resorption in the dams and of cleft palates in the pups. Susceptibility of dams to cleft palate in offspring was greatest on days 12-15 of gestation (Steffek *et al.*, 1972).

Semicarbazide hydrochloride binds to cytosine residues in RNA, to deoxycytosine residues in DNA *in vitro* and to cytosine and deoxycytosine nucleosides (Hayatsu & Ukita, 1966; Hayatsu *et al.*, 1966).

(b) Man

No data were available to the Working Group.

3.3 Case reports and epidemiological studies

No data were available to the Working Group.

4. Comments on Data Reported and Evaluation[1]

4.1 Animal data

Semicarbazide hydrochloride is carcinogenic in mice after its oral administration: it produced angiomas, angiosarcomas and lung tumours.

---

[1]See also the section, 'Animal data in relation to the evaluation of risk to man' in the introduction to this volume, p. 13.

4.2 Human data

No case reports or epidemiological studies were available to the Working Group.

5. References

Grasselli, J.G., ed. (1973) Atlas of Spectral Data and Physical Constants for Organic Compounds, Cleveland, Ohio, Chemical Rubber Co., p. B-891

Hawley, G.G., ed. (1971) Condensed Chemical Dictionary, 8th ed., New York, Van Nostrand-Reinhold, p. 779

Hayatsu, H. & Ukita, T. (1966) Modification of nucleosides and nucleotides. IV. Reaction of semicarbazide with nucleic acids. Biochim. biophys. acta, 123, 458-470

Hayatsu, H., Takeishi, K.I. & Ukita, T. (1966) Modification of nucleosides and nucleotides. III. A selective modification of cytidine with semicarbazide. Biochim. biophys. acta, 123, 445-457

IARC (1974) IARC Monographs on the Evaluation of Carcinogenic Risk of Chemicals to Man, 4, Some Aromatic Amines, Hydrazine and Related Substances, N-Nitroso Compounds and Miscellaneous Alkylating Agents, Lyon, pp. 127-136

Jenney, E.H. & Pfeiffer, C.C. (1958) The convulsant effect of hydrazides and the antidotal effect of anticonvulsants and metabolites. J. Pharmacol. exp. Ther., 122, 110-123

Korczynski, A. (1969) Continuous electrochemical production of semicarbazide hydrochloride. Zesz. Nauk. Politech. Slask., Chem., 50, 189-191

Mori, K., Yasuno, A. & Matsumoto, K. (1960) Induction of pulmonary tumors in mice with isonicotinic acid hydrazid. Gann, 51, 83-89

Pszonicka, M. & Skwara, W. (1970) The use of Co(III)solutions in acetic acid for oxidimetric titrations. IV. Potentiometric determination of some derivatives of hydrazine, ascorbic acid and cysteine. Chem. analyt. (Warsaw), 15, 175-182

Stecher, P.G., ed. (1968) The Merck Index, 8th ed., Rahway, NJ, Merck & Co., p. 941

Steffek, A.J., Verrusio, A.C. & Watkins, C.A. (1972) Cleft palate in rodents after maternal treatment with various lathyrogenic agents. Teratology, 5, 33-40

Stivers, F.E., Steffek, A.J. & Yarington, C.T., Jr (1971) Effect of lathyrogens on developing mid-facial structures in the rat. J. surg. Res., 11, 415-420

Thiele, J. & Stange, O. (1894) Über Semicarbazid. Chem. Ber., 27, 31-34

Toth, B. & Shimizu, H. (1974) 1-Carbamyl-2-phenylhydrazine tumorigenesis in Swiss mice. Morphology of lung adenomas. J. nat. Cancer Inst., 52, 241-251

Toth, B., Shimizu, H. & Erickson, J. (1975) Carbamylhydrazine hydrochloride as a lung and blood vessel tumour inducer in Swiss mice. Europ. J. Cancer, 11, 17-22

Ulland, B., Weisburger, E.K. & Weisburger, J.H. (1973) Chronic toxicity and carcinogenicity of industrial chemicals and pesticides. Toxicol. appl. Pharmacol., 25, 446

US International Trade Commission (1975) Synthetic Organic Chemicals, US Production and Sales, 1973, ITC Publication 728, Washington DC, US Government Printing Office, p. 218

US Tariff Commission (1941) Synthetic Organic Chemicals, US Production and Sales, 1940, Report No. 148, Second Series, Washington DC, US Government Printing Office, p. 57

Weast, R.C., ed. (1975) CRC Handbook of Chemistry and Physics, 56th ed., Cleveland, Ohio, Chemical Rubber Co., p. C-489

SODIUM DIETHYLDITHIOCARBAMATE

1. Chemical and Physical Data

1.1 Synonyms and trade names

Chem. Abstr. Reg. Serial No.: 148-18-5

Chem. Abstr. Name: Diethylcarbamodithioic acid, sodium salt

DEDC; diethyldithiocarbamate sodium; diethyldithiocarbamic acid sodium salt; N,N-diethyldithiocarbamic acid, sodium salt; diethyl sodium dithiocarbamate; dithiocarb; sodium DEDT; sodium N,N-diethyldithiocarbamic acid; sodium salt of N,N-diethyldithiocarbamic acid

1.2 Chemical formula and molecular weight

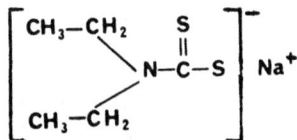

$$\left[\begin{array}{c} \text{CH}_3\text{--CH}_2 \\ \\ \text{CH}_3\text{--CH}_2 \end{array} \!\!\! \begin{array}{c} \text{S} \\ \| \\ \text{N--C--S} \end{array} \right]^{-} \text{Na}^{+}$$

$C_5H_{10}NNaS_2$ Mol. wt: 171.3

1.3 Chemical and physical properties of the substance

From Stecher (1968), unless otherwise specified

(a) Description: Platelets (Koch, 1949)

(b) Melting-point: 94-96°C

(c) Spectroscopy data: λ_{max} = 257 nm and 290 nm (E^1_1 = 700 and 760) (Koch, 1949)

(d) Solubility: Freely soluble in water at room temperature; soluble in ethanol

(e) Stability: Aqueous solutions decompose slowly.

1.4 Technical products and impurities

Sodium diethyldithiocarbamate is available in the US for use in rubber processing as a 25% active aqueous solution, with, typically, a pale yellow colour and a density of 1.08-1.10 (Anon., 1975).

2. Production, Use, Occurrence and Analysis

For important background information on this section, see preamble, p. 15.

2.1 Production and use

The first reported preparation of sodium diethyldithiocarbamate was by the addition of carbon disulphide to an aqueous solution of diethylamine and sodium hydroxide (Delepine, 1907). The same method is believed to be used for its commercial production (Tisdale & Williams, 1934).

Commercial production of sodium diethyldithiocarbamate was first reported in the US in 1940 (US Tariff Commission, 1941). In 1969, three manufacturers reported sales of 65 thousand kg (US Tariff Commission, 1971). In 1974, one manufacturer reported production (US International Trade Commission, 1975).

It is estimated that less than 1 million kg sodium diethyldithio-carbamate are produced annually in Austria, the Benelux countries, France, the Federal Republic of Germany, Italy and the UK.

This compound is used in the rubber-processing industry as a latex accelerator (Anon., 1975). It is also used as a chemical intermediate in the production of other diethyldithiocarbamate metal salts, such as the zinc, selenium and tellurium salts, and of bis(thiocarbamoyl)sulphides, which are used as rubber-processing accelerators and fungicides (Shaver, 1968). It is used to separate copper from other metals (Stecher, 1968); other miscellaneous applications include its use as an oxidation inhibitor (Hawley, 1971), a chelating agent and as an analytical reagent (Stecher, 1968). It has been used as a chelating agent in human therapy, for the treatment of nickel carbonyl poisoning (Sunderman, 1964).

2.2 Occurrence

Sodium diethyldithiocarbamate is not known to occur as a natural product.

2.3 Analysis

Concentrations of $5 \times 10^{-5} - 8 \times 10^{-4}$ M dithiocarbamates have been analysed by direct-current polarographic methods in which anodic waves correspond to the formation of mercury compounds (Halls *et al.*, 1968); when short, controlled drop times are used, concentrations of 1.6×10^{-3} M can be determined by this method (Canterford *et al.*, 1973). The application of differential pulse polarography has increased the sensitivity of the method to a detection limit of 1×10^{-6} M and a quantitative limit of 2×10^{-6} M (Canterford & Buchanan, 1973).

Sodium diethyldithiocarbamate can be determined by titration of the excess iodine solution resulting from the sodium diethyldithiocarbamate-induced iodine-azide reaction. The range which could be determined was from 5-160 μg in 50 or 100 cm^3 of solution, with a relative error of ±3% (Kurzawa & Kubaszewski, 1974).

A thin-layer chromatographic-spectrofluorimetric method (van Hoof & Heyndrickz, 1973) is suitable for the analysis of a variety of metal dithiocarbamates, although it was not applied to sodium diethyldithiocarbamate itself.

3. Biological Data Relevant to the Evaluation of Carcinogenic Risk to Man

3.1 Carcinogenicity and related studies in animals

(a) Oral administration

Mouse: Groups of 18 male and 18 female (C57BL/6xC3H/Anf)F_1 mice and 18 male and 18 female (C57BL/6xAKR)F_1 mice received sodium diethyldithiocarbamate (m.p. 94-96°C) according to the following schedule: 215 mg/kg bw in water at 7 days of age by stomach tube and the same amount (not adjusted for increasing body weight) daily up to 4 weeks of age; subsequently, the mice were given 692 mg sodium diethyldithiocarbamate per kg of diet. The dose was the maximum tolerated dose for infant and young mice but not necessarily so for adults. The experiment was terminated when the animals were about 78 weeks of age, at which time 17, 18, 18 and 16 mice in the four groups, respectively, were still alive. Tumour incidences were compared with those in 79-90 necropsied mice of each sex and strain, which either had been untreated or had received gelatine. Pulmonary adenomas occurred in 3/17 [P>0.05] and 5/18 [P<0.05] males of the two strains, respectively, compared with 5/79 and 9/90 in controls. Hepatomas developed in 7/17 males of the first strain, compared with 8/79 in control males [P<0.01]. There was no increase in the incidence of liver tumours among males of the other strain, and no liver tumours occurred in females (Innes *et al.*, 1969; NTIS, 1968).

(b) Subcutaneous administration

Mouse: Groups of 18 male and 18 female (C57BL/6xC3H/Anf)F_1 mice and 18 male and 18 female (C57BL/6xAKR)F_1 mice were given single s.c. injections of 464 mg/kg bw sodium diethyldithiocarbamate (m.p. 94-96°C) in water on the 28th day of life and were observed until they were about 78 weeks of age, at which time 16, 18, 18 and 16 mice in the four groups, respectively, were still alive. Tumour incidences were compared with those in groups of 141, 154, 161 and 157 untreated or vehicle-injected controls that were necropsied. Incidences were not increased (P>0.05) for any tumour type in any sex-strain subgroup or in the combined sexes of either strain (NTIS, 1968) [The Working Group noted that a negative result obtained with a single s.c. injection may not be an adequate basis for discounting carcinogenicity].

3.2 Other relevant biological data

(a) Experimental systems

The i.p. LD_{50} of sodium diethyldithiocarbamate in mice is about 1 g/kg bw (Maj & Vetulani, 1970). In a 6-week experiment in mice, daily s.c. injections of 50 mg/kg bw had marked anti-thyroid activity (Ambrus *et al.*, 1951).

In rats, four metabolites, diethyldithiocarbamate, diethyldithiocarba-mate-S-glucuronide, inorganic sulphate and carbon disulphide were identified; these are also metabolites of disulfiram (Strömme, 1965).

Sodium diethyldithiocarbamate reduces blood copper concentrations. Pregnant rabbits injected intravenously with 0.5 g sodium diethyldithiocar-bamate/day on 5 days per week throughout pregnancy failed to deliver litters (Howell, 1964).

A small but significant increase in the number of chromosome breakages and aberrations was found in *Vicia faba* (Kihlman, 1957).

(b) Man

Sodium diethyldithiocarbamate has been used in the treatment of 13 cases of acute nickel carbonyl poisoning and in one case of hepatolenti-cular degeneration (Wilson's disease) (Sunderman, 1964).

3.3 Case reports and epidemiological studies

No data were available to the Working Group.

4. Comments on Data Reported and Evaluation

4.1 Animal data

Sodium diethyldithiocarbamate has been tested by oral administration and by single subcutaneous injection in two strains of mice. Although it produced an increase in the incidence of liver-cell tumours in males of one strain and a slight increase of lung tumours in males of the other strain following its oral administration, the available data are insufficient to make an evaluation of the carcinogenicity of this compound.

4.2 Human data

No case reports or epidemiological studies were available to the Working Group.

5. References

Ambrus, C.M., Ambrus, J.L. & Harrisson, J.W.E. (1951) Effect of sodium diethyldithiocarbamate on thyroid activity. Amer. J. Pharmacol., 123, 129-130

Anon. (1975) Materials and Compounding Ingredients for Rubber, New York, Bill Communications, p. 45

Canterford, D.R. & Buchanan, A.S. (1973) Application of differential pulse polarography to anodic electrode processes involving mercury compound formation. Electroanalyt. Chem. Interfacial Electrochem., 44, 291-298

Canterford, D.R., Buchanan, A.S. & Bond, A.M. (1973) Advantages of rapid direct current polarography in the presence of analytically undesirable phenomena associated with anodic mercury waves. Analyt. Chem., 45, 1327-1331

Delepine, M. (1907) Metallic salts of dithiocarbamic acids; preparation of isothiocyanates in the aliphatic series. C.R. Acad. Sci. (Paris), 144, 1125-1127

Halls, D.J., Townshend, A. & Zuman, P. (1968) Polarography of some sulphur-containing compounds. XIII. Anodic waves of dialkyldithiocarbamates. Analyt. chim. acta, 41, 51-62

Hawley, G.G., ed. (1971) Condensed Chemical Dictionary, 8th ed., New York, Van Nostrand-Reinhold, p. 799

van Hoof, F. & Heyndrickx, A. (1973) Thin layer chromatographic-spectro-photophuorimetric methods for the determination of dithio- and thiol-carbamates after hydrolysis and coupling with NBD-Cl. Ghent. Rijks-univ. Fac. Landbl. Med., 38, 911-916

Howell, J.M. (1964) Effect of sodium diethyldithiocarbamate on blood copper-levels and pregnancy in the rabbit. Nature (Lond.), 201, 83-84

Innes, J.R.M., Ulland, B.M, Valerio, M.G., Petrucelli, L., Fishbein, L., Hart, E.R., Pallotta, A.J., Bates, R.R., Falk, H.L., Gart, J.J., Klein, M., Mitchell, I. & Peters, J. (1969) Bioassay of pesticides and industrial chemicals for tumorigenicity in mice: a preliminary note. J. nat. Cancer Inst., 42, 1101-1114

Kihlman, B.A. (1957) Experimentally induced chromosome aberrations in plants. I. The production of chromosome aberrations by cyanide and other heavy metal complexing agents. J. biophys. biochem. Cytol., 3, 363-380

Koch, H.P. (1949) Absorption spectra and structure of organic sulphur compounds. III. Vulcanisation accelerators and related compounds. J. chem. Soc., 401-408

Kurzawa, Z. & Kubaszewski, E. (1974) Determination of microgram amounts of sodium diethyldithiocarbamate by means of iodine-azide reaction. Chem. analyt. (Warsaw), 19, 263-269

Maj, J. & Vetulani, J. (1970) Some pharmacological properties of N,N-disubstituted dithiocarbamates and their effect on the brain catecholamine levels. Europ. J. Pharmacol., 9, 183-189

NTIS (National Technical Information Service) (1968) Evaluation of Carcinogenic, Teratogenic and Mutagenic Activities of Selected Pesticides and Industrial Chemicals, Vol. 1, Carcinogenic Study, Washington DC, US Department of Commerce

Shaver, F.W. (1968) Rubber chemicals. In: Kirk, R.E. & Othmer, D.F., eds, Encyclopedia of Chemical Technology, 2nd ed., Vol. 17, New York, John Wiley & Sons, pp. 513-514

Stecher, P.G., ed. (1968) The Merck Index, 8th ed., Rahway, NJ, Merck & Co., p. 958

Strömme, J.H. (1965) Metabolism of disulfiram and diethyldithiocarbamate in rats with demonstration of an *in vivo* ethanol-induced inhibition of the glucuronic acid conjugation of the thiol. Biochem. Pharmacol., 14, 393-410

Sunderman, F.W. (1964) Nickel and copper mobilization by sodium diethyl-dithiocarbamate. J. New Drugs, May-June, 154-161

Tisdale, W.H. & Williams, I. (1934) Disinfectant. US Patent 1,972,961, September 11, to E.I. du Pont de Nemours & Co.

US International Trade Commission (1975) Synthetic Organic Chemicals, US Production and Sales of Rubber-Processing Chemicals, 1974 Preliminary, Washington DC, US Government Printing Office, p. 7

US Tariff Commission (1941) Synthetic Organic Chemicals, US Production and Sales, 1940, Report No. 148, Second Series, Washington DC, US Government Printing Office, p. 50

US Tariff Commission (1971) Synthetic Organic Chemicals, US Production and Sales, 1969, TC Publication No. 412, Washington DC, US Government Printing Office, pp. 144, 148-149

THIRAM

1. Chemical and Physical Data

1.1 Synonyms and trade names

Chem. Abstr. Reg. Serial No.: 137-26-8

Chem. Abstr. Name: Tetramethylthioperoxydicarbonic diamide

Bis[(dimethylamino)carbonothioyl] disulphide; bis(dimethylthiocarbamoyl) disulphide; bis(*N*,*N*-dimethylthiocarbamoyl) disulphide; bis(dimethyl-thiocarbamyl) disulphide; 1,1'-dithiobis(*N*,*N*-dimethylthioformamide); α,α-dithiobis(dimethylthio)formamide; α,α'-dithiobis(dimethyl-thio)formamide; *N*,*N*'-(dithiodicarbonothioyl)bis(*N*-methylmethanamine); methyl thiram; methyl thiuramdisulphide; tetramethyldiurane: I sulphite; tetramethylenethiuram disulphide; tetramethylthio-carbamoyldisulphide; tetramethylthiuram; tetramethylthiuram bisul-phide; tetramethyl thiuram disulphide; *N*,*N*'-tetramethylthiuram disulphide; *N*,*N*,*N*',*N*'-tetramethylthiuram disulphide; tetramethyl-thiuran disulphide; tetramethyl thiurane disulphide; tetramethyl-thiurum disulphide; tetrathiuram disulphide; thiuram; TMTD; TMTDS

Accelerator Thiuram; Aceto TETD; Arasan; Arasan 42-S; Arasan 70; Arasan 75; Arasan-M; Arasan-SF; Cyuram DS; Ekagom TB; Fernasan; Fernasan A; Fernide; Hermal; Heryl; Kregasan; Mercuram; Methyl Tuads; Nobecutan; Nomersan; Panoram 75; Polyram Ultra; Pomarsol; Pomarsol Forte; Pomasol; Puralin; Rezifilm; Royal TMTD; Sadoplon; Spotrete; Tersan; Tetrasipton; Thillate; Thiosan; Thiotox; Thiram B; Thiram 75; Thirasan; Thiulin; Thiurad; Thiuram D; Thiuram M; Thiuram M Rubber Accelerator; Thiuramyl; Thuiram; Thylate; Tiuramyl; Tridipam; Tripomol; Tuads; Tuex; Tulisan; VUAgt-I-4; Vulcafor TMTD; Vulkacit MTIC

1.2 Chemical formula and molecular weight

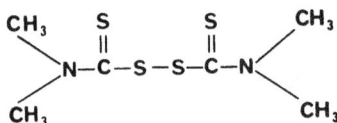

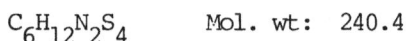

$$CH_3\!-\!N\overset{\underset{\displaystyle CH_3}{|}}{\,}\!-\!\overset{\overset{\displaystyle S}{\|}}{C}\!-\!S\!-\!S\!-\!\overset{\overset{\displaystyle S}{\|}}{C}\!-\!N\overset{\underset{\displaystyle CH_3}{|}}{\,}\!-\!CH_3$$

$$C_6H_{12}N_2S_4 \qquad \text{Mol. wt: } 240.4$$

1.3 Chemical and physical properties of the substance

From Weast (1975), unless otherwise specified

(a) Description: White or yellow monoclinic crystals

(b) Boiling-point: 129°C at 20 mm

(c) Melting-point: 155-156°C

(d) Spectroscopy data: λ_{max} 243 nm (in chloroform) and 282 nm
(E_1^1 = 478 and 524); for infra-red and nuclear magnetic resonance
spectral data, see Grasselli (1973)

(e) Solubility: Insoluble in water, alkalis and aliphatic hydrocarbons; slightly soluble in ethanol and ether (<0.2%);
soluble in acetone (1.2%), benzene (2.5%) and chloroform
(Stecher, 1968)

(f) Stability: Decomposed by acids (Association of American
Pesticide Control Officials, Inc., 1962)

1.4 Technical products and impurities

Thiram powder is available commercially in the US with the following
specifications: white to cream powder; density, 1.42±0.03; melting-range,
142-156°C; moisture, 1.0% max.; ash, 0.5% max.; particle size, 99.9%
passes through a 100-mesh screen; petroleum ether extract, 1.0-3.0% (Anon.,
1974).

For rubber processing, thiram is available as a fine powder containing
1.5-2.5% (max.) white oil, as extruded pellets containing 5.5% oil, as a
dispersion containing 30-40% binder or oil, in a mixture of two parts
thiram to one part 2-mercaptobenzothiazole, and as pellets in a 50:50

mixture with disulfiram (Anon., 1975).

For use as a pesticide, thiram is available as 1.0-75.0% in dust; as 2.25-5.0% in granules; as 11.25, 35.2, and 42.0% in liquid concentrates; as 2.0% in paste; as 1.0% in paints for wound dressing of shrubs and trees; and as 3.0-98.0% in wettable powders (US Environmental Protection Agency, 1974).

Specifications for this product in Japan are: purity, 98%; appearance, yellow powder; melting-point, above 103°C; water, less than 0.3%; unspecified inorganic impurities, 0.3%; and organic impurities [bis(dimethyldithiocarbamoyl)sulphide and bis(pentamethylene thiocarbamoyl)tetrasulphide], 1.0 to 1.4% (Japanese Ministry of Agriculture and Forestry, 1975).

2. Production, Use, Occurrence and Analysis

For important background information on this section, see preamble, p. 15.

2.1 Production and use

Thiram was first prepared by the oxidation of the dimethylamine salt of dimethyldithiocarbamic acid with iodine in an ethanolic solution (von Braun, 1902). Although several other methods have been described, thiram is believed to be produced commercially in the US by passing chlorine gas through a solution of sodium dimethyldithiocarbamate (Wenyon, 1972). In Canada, it is produced commercially by the oxidation of sodium dimethyldithiocarbamate with hydrogen peroxide or iodine (Spencer, 1973). In Japan, it is produced commercially from iron oxide, hydrogen peroxide, sodium hydroxide, dimethylamine and carbon disulphide (Japanese Ministry of Agriculture and Forestry, 1975).

Thiram was first produced commercially in the US in 1925 (US Tariff Commission, 1926); production was 2 million kg in 1960 (US Tariff Commission, 1961) and 7.9 million kg in 1973 (US International Trade Commission, 1975a). In 1974, four US companies reported the production of 5.8 million kg (US International Trade Commission, 1975b).

It is estimated that total annual production of thiram in Europe is from 5 to 10 million kg, produced in the Benelux countries, France, the Federal Republic of Germany, Italy, Spain and the UK. In Japan, commercial production of thiram began in 1953. In 1970, four companies reported the production of 140 thousand kg, and in 1974, 238 thousand kg (Japanese Ministry of Agriculture and Forestry, 1975).

About 97% of the thiram utilized in the US is as primary and secondary accelerators in compounding natural, isobutylene-isoprene, butadiene, styrene-butadiene, synthetic isoprene and nitrile-butadiene rubbers. It renders low sulphur and sulphur-less stock heat-resistant, is non-discolouring and non-staining, and is an excellent activator for guanidines, amines and thiazoles. Thiram is also used as a cure retarder in Neoprene G rubbers (Anon., 1975).

It is also used as a fungicide on seeds, fruits, nuts, vegetables and ornamental crops, and on paper, polyurethane foam products and industrial textiles (US Environmental Protection Agency, 1974). It is used as an animal repellant, to protect trees and shrubs from rabbit and deer depredation (Berg, 1975). Thiram may have been used as a bacteriostat in soap (Klarmann, 1963) and antiseptic sprays (Stecher, 1968). Miscellaneous applications include its use as an anti-oxidant in polyolefin plastics (Dugan, 1963) and as a peptizing agent in polysulphide elastomers (Saltman, 1965).

According to the US Occupational Safety and Health administration health standards for air contaminants, an employee's exposure to thiram should not exceed 5 mg/m^3 in the workplace air during any eight-hour workshift for a forty-hour work week (US Code of Federal Regulations, 1975). The maximum allowable concentration proposed in the USSR is 0.5 mg/m^3 (Winell, 1975).

In the US, residue tolerances for thiram when used as a fungicide were set at levels of up to 7 mg/kg for a variety of fruits and vegetables. Restrictions were also placed on the use of treated seeds (US Environmental Protection Agency, 1974).

In December 1974, the Joint Meeting of the FAO Working Party of Experts on Pesticide Residues and the WHO Expert Committee on Pesticide Residues established a revised temporary acceptable daily intake for man of 0-0.005 mg/kg bw for all dimethyldithiocarbamate fungicides (WHO, 1975a,b).

2.2 Occurrence

Thiram is not known to occur as a natural product. Residual amounts may rest on or in treated crops after harvesting.

2.3 Analysis

A method for the quantitative determination of thiram in vegetables, based on gas-chromatographic analysis of the carbon disulphide evolved was used for determinations in samples containing 3.5 and 7.0 mg/kg (McLeod & McCully, 1969). A microbiological method using *Saccharomyces carlsbergensis* ATCC 9080 as the test organism has been developed for the determination of thiram in food preparations; as little as 25 ng/well or 200 ng/disc can be detected on agar plates (Rappe *et al.*, 1973).

Gel permeation and thin-layer chromatographic methods were used for the analysis of vulcanization accelerators, including thiram, in extracts of synthetic rubbers and mixtures of technical rubber additives (Protivová *et al.*, 1974). A thin-layer chromatographic-spectrophotofluorimetric method for the estimation of thiram allows detection of 40 ng (van Hoof & Heyndrickx, 1973).

3. Biological Data Relevant to the Evaluation of Carcinogenic Risk to Man

3.1 Carcinogenicity and related studies in animals

(a) Oral administration

Mouse: Groups of 18 male and 18 female (C57BL/6xC3H/Anf)F_1 mice and 18 male and 18 female (C57BL/6xAKR)F_1 mice received commercial thiram (m.p. 154-156°C) according to the following schedule: 10 mg/kg bw in gelatine at 7 days of age by stomach tube and the same amount (not adjusted for increasing body weight) daily up to 4 weeks of age; subsequently, the mice were given 26 mg thiram per kg of diet. The dose given was the maximum tolerated dose for infant and young mice but not necessarily so for

adults. The experiment was terminated when the animals were about 78 weeks
of age, at which time 16, 18, 18 and 15 mice in the four groups, respectively,
were still alive. Tumour incidences were compared with those observed among
79-90 necropsied mice of each sex and strain, which either had been untreated
or had received gelatine only: the incidences were not significantly greater
(P>0.05) for any tumour type in any sex-strain subgroup or in the combined
sexes of either strain (Innes et al., 1969; NTIS, 1968).

An unspecified number of C57BL mice were given weekly doses of 300 mg/kg
bw thiram by stomach tube for 5 weeks and were killed at intervals of up to
9 months after the last dose. Of 51 mice killed at 9 months, 2 had lung
adenomas. The incidence in untreated controls is not given (Chernov
et al., 1972) [The short duration of this experiment should be noted].

(b) Subcutaneous administration

Mouse: Groups of 18 male and 18 female (C57BL/6xC3H/Anf)F_1 mice and
18 male and 18 female (C57BL/6xAKR)F_1 mice were given single s.c. injections
of 46.4 mg/kg bw thiram (m.p. 154-156°C) in 0.5% gelatine on the 28th day
of life and were observed until they were about 78 weeks of age, at which
time 16, 16, 17 and 16 mice in the four groups, respectively, were still
alive. Tumour incidences were compared with those in groups of 141, 154,
161 and 157 untreated or vehicle-injected controls that were necropsied.
Incidences were not increased (P>0.05) for any tumour type in any sex-strain
subgroup or in the combined sexes of either strain (NTIS, 1968) [The Working
Group noted that a negative result obtained with a single s.c. injection
may not be an adequate basis for discounting carcinogenicity].

3.2 Other relevant biological data

(a) Experimental systems

The approximate oral LD_{50} values for thiram in mice, rats and rabbits
are 1800, 820 and 210 mg/kg bw, respectively (Kirchheim, 1951; Lehman, 1951).
An oral LD_{50} of 2300 mg/kg bw has been reported in virgin female NMRI strain
mice (Matthiaschk, 1973). The dermal LD_{50} in rats is more than 2000 mg/kg bw
(Ben-Dyke et al., 1970).

230

No adverse effects were seen in a 3-generation study in which rats were fed 48 mg thiram per kg of diet. In rats fed diets containing 100, 300 or 500 mg per kg of diet for 2 years, there were small reductions in growth rates; among those fed the two higher levels there was increased mortality; and in those at the highest dose there were convulsions, thyroid hyperplasia (Griepentrog, 1962) and calcification of the cerebellum, hypothalamus and medulla oblongata (WHO, 1965).

Like most dithiocarbamates, thiram induces the accumulation of acetaldehyde in the blood of rats receiving ethanol at the same time (van Logten, 1972). Its reaction with nitrite at an acid pH in the stomachs of guinea-pigs *in vivo* gives rise to N-nitrosodimethylamine (Elespuru & Lijinsky, 1973; Sen *et al.*, 1974).

When pregnant NMRI mice were given oral doses of 10-30 mg/animal from day 5-15 of pregancy, increased resorption occurred during intermediate and late stages of foetogenesis. Malformations, characterized by cleft palates, micrognathia, wavy ribs and distorted bones, were found in the developing foetuses and in the pups at term (Matthiaschk, 1973; Roll, 1971). Simultaneous administration of thiram and 10 mg/animal L-cysteine intraperitoneally from day 5-15 of pregnancy resulted in a significant decrease both in the severity and in the number of embryopathies (Matthiaschk, 1973).

Thiram induced chromosome aberrations in barley (George *et al.*, 1970), but no increase in the number of chlorophyll mutations was found in wheat (Mamalyga *et al.*, 1974). An increased number of chromosomal aberrations was observed in metaphases of bone-marrow cells of mice treated with 100 mg/kg bw orally (Antonovich *et al.*, 1971).

(b) Man

Doses of 0.5 g/day have been taken for several weeks without adverse effects, provided that no ethanol was consumed (Domingo, 1952). For a discussion of the interaction of compounds such as thiram with ethanol in the blood, see 'General Remarks on Carbamates, Thiocarbamates and Carbazides', pp. 28-29.

3.3 Case reports and epidemiological studies

In a group of 223 workers (42 men and 181 women), mostly aged between 20-50 years, engaged in the manufacture of thiram for more than 3 years and observed for several years subsequently, various clinical and pathological manifestations, including ocular irritation, coughing, thoracic pain, tachicardia, epistaxis, dermal lesions, myocardiodystrophia, clinical and subclinical liver dysfunction and asthenia were reported, often in excess of those seen in a group of 193 persons not in contact with thiram. Enlargement of the thyroid gland was more common in the exposed group. One case of adenocarcinoma of the thyroid and 7 others with thyroid abnormalities were reported among 105 workers examined (Cherpak *et al.*, 1971; Kaskevich & Bezugly, 1973).

4. Comments on Data Reported and Evaluation

4.1 Animal data

Thiram has been tested by oral administration and by single subcutaneous injection in mice. Although no carcinogenic effect was observed in these studies, the available data are insufficient for an evaluation of the carcinogenicity of this compound to be made.

Thiram can react with nitrite under mildly acid conditions, simulating those in the human stomach, to form *N*-nitrosodimethylamine, which has been shown to be carcinogenic in seven animal species (IARC, 1972).

4.2 Human data

The one case of thyroid cancer reported forms an insufficient basis on which to evaluate the carcinogenicity of thiram in man.

5. References

Anon. (1974) Methyl Tuads®, New York, R.T. Vanderbilt Co.

Anon. (1975) Materials and Compounding Ingredients for Rubber, New York, Bill Communications, pp. 31-59

Antonovich, E.A., Chepynoga, O.P., Chernov, O.V., Rjazanova, P.A., Vekshtein, M.S., Martson, V.S., Martson, L.V., Samosh, L.V., Pilinskaya, M.A., Kurinny, L.I., Balin, P.N., Khitsenko, I.I., Zastavnjuk, N.P. & Zaolorozhnaja, N.A. (1971) Toxicity of dithiocarbamates and their fate in warmblooded animals. In: Antonovich, E.A., Bojanovska, A., Engst, P. *et al.*, eds, Proceedings of the Symposium on Toxicology and Analytical Chemistry of Dithiocarbamates, Dubrovnic, 1970, Beograd, pp. 3-20

Association of American Pesticide Control Officials, Inc. (1962) Pesticide Chemicals Official Compendium, Box HH, University P.O., College Park, Maryland, p. 307

Ben-Dyke, R., Sanderson, D.M. & Noakes, D.N. (1970) Acute toxicity data for pesticides. Wld Rev. Pest. Control, 9, 119-127

Berg, G.L., ed. (1975) Farm Chemicals Handbook 1975, Willoughby, Ohio, Meister, p. D 203

von Braun, J. (1902) Thiuramdisulfides and iso-thiuramdisulfides. I. Chem. Ber., 35, 817-829

Chernov, O.V., Khitsenko, I.I. & Balin, P.N. (1972) Blastomogenic properties of some derivatives of dithiocarbamic acid and their metabolites. Onkologiya, 3, 123-126

Cherpak, V.V., Bezugly, V.P. & Kaskevich, L.M. (1971) Sanitary-hygienic characteristics of working conditions and health of persons working with tetramethylthiuram disulfide (TMTD). Vrach. Delo, 10, 136-139

Domingo, A.F. (1952) Ensayos de toxicidad con maiz tratados con 'Arasan' y 'Spergon'. Rev. Med. Vet. (Caracas), 11, 335-348

Dugan, L.R. (1963) Antioxidants. In: Kirk, R.E. & Othmer, D.F., eds, Encyclopedia of Chemical Technology, 2nd ed., Vol. 2, New York, John Wiley & Sons, pp. 600-604

Elespuru, R.K. & Lijinsky, W. (1973) The formation of carcinogenic nitroso compounds from nitrite and some types of agricultural chemicals. Fd Cosmet. Toxicol., 11, 807-817

George, M.K., Aulakh, K.S. & Dhesi, J.S. (1970) Morphological and cytological changes induced in barley (*Hordeum vulgare*) seedlings following seed treatment with fungicides. Canad. J. Genet. Cytol., 12, 415-419

233

Grasselli, J.G., ed. (1973) Atlas of Spectral Data and Physical Constants for Organic Compounds, Cleveland, Ohio, Chemical Rubber Co., p. B-484

Griepentrog, F. (1962) Tumorartige Schilddrüsenveränderungen in chronisch-toxikologischen Tierversuchen mit Thiuramen. Beitr. Path. Anat., 126, 243-255

van Hoof, F. & Heyndrickx, A. (1973) Thin layer chromatographic-spectro-photo uorimetric methods for the determination of dithio- and thiol-carbamates after hydrolysis and coupling with NBD-Cl. Ghent. Rijks-univ. Fac. Landbl. Med., 38, 911-916

IARC (1972) IARC Monographs on the Evaluation of Carcinogenic Risk of Chemicals to Man, 1, Lyon, pp. 95-106

Innes, J.R.M., Ulland, B.M., Valerio, M.G., Petrucelli, L., Fishbein, L., Hart, E.R., Pallotta, A.J., Bates, R.R., Falk, H.L., Gart, J.J., Klein, M., Mitchell, I. & Peters, J. (1969) Bioassay of pesticides and industrial chemicals for tumorigenicity in mice: a preliminary note. J. nat. Cancer Inst., 42, 1101-1114

Japanese Ministry of Agriculture and Forestry (1975) Noyaku Yoran (Agri-cultural Chemicals Annual), 1975, Division of Plant Disease Prevention, Tokyo, Takeo Endo, pp. 17-20, 22, 26, 86, 89, 101, 254, 267-269, 271, 275, 301

Kaskevich, L.M. & Bezugly, V.P. (1973) Clinical aspects of intoxications induced by TMTD. Vrach. Delo, 6, 128-130

Kirchheim, D. (1951) Toxizität und Wirkung einiger Thiuramdisulfid-verbindungen auf den Alkoholstoffwechsel. Naunyn-Schmiedeberg's Arch. exp. Path. Pharmakol., 214, 59-66

Klarmann, E.G. (1963) Antiseptics and disinfectants. In: Kirk, R.E. & Othmer, D.F., eds, Encylopedia of Chemical Technology, 2nd ed., Vol. 2, New York, John Wiley & Sons, pp. 636-637

Lehman, A.J. (1951) Chemicals in food: a report of the association of food and drug officials on current developments. II. Pesticides. Quart. Bull. Ass. Fd Drug Off. US, 15, 122-133

van Logten, M.J. (1972) De Dithiocarbamaat-Alcohol-Reactie bij de Rat, Terborg, The Netherlands, Bedrijf FA. Lammers, p. 38

Mamalyga, V.S., Kulik, M.I. & Logvinenko, V.F. (1974) Induced chlorophyll mutations in hard spring wheat. Dokl. Akad. Nauk SSSR, 215, 211-213

Matthiaschk, G. (1973) Über den Einfluss von L-cystein auf die Teratogenese durch Thiram (TMTD) bei NMRI-Mäusen. Arch. Toxikol., 30, 251-262

McLeod, H.A. & McCully, K.A. (1969) Head space gas procedure for screening food samples for dithiocarbamate pesticide residues. J. Ass. off. analyt. Chem., 52, 1226-1230

NTIS (National Technical Information Service) (1968) Evaluation of Carcino-genic, Teratogenic and Mutagenic Activities of Selected Pesticides and Industrial Chemicals, Vol. 1, Carcinogenic Study, Washington DC, US Department of Commerce

Protivova, J., Pospisil, J. & Holcik, J. (1974) Antioxidants and stabilizers. XLVIII. Analysis of the components of stabilization and vulcanization mixtures for rubbers by gel permeation and thin-layer chromatographic methods. J. Chromat., 92, 361-370

Rappe, A., Mauquoy, G. & Bauer, S. (1973) Microbiological determination of thiram. J. Ass. off. analyt. Chem., 56, 1517-1518

Reinl, W. (1966) Alkoholüberempfindlichkeit nach Umgang mit dem Fungicid Tetramethylthiuramdisulfid (TMTD). Arch. Toxikol., 22, 12-15

Roll, R. (1971) Teratologische Untersuchungen mit Thiram (TMTD) an zwei Mäusestämmen. Arch. Toxikol., 27, 173-186

Saltman, W.M. (1965) Elastomers, synthetic. In: Kirk, R.E. & Othmer, D.F., eds, Encyclopedia of Chemical Technology, 2nd ed., Vol. 7, New York, John Wiley & Sons, pp. 696-697

Sen, N.P., Donaldson, B.A. & Charbonneau, C. (1974) Formation of nitroso-dimethylamine from the interaction of certain pesticides and nitrites. In: Bogovski, P. & Walker, E.A., eds, N-Nitroso Compounds in the Environment, Lyon, IARC (IARC Scientific Publications No. 9), pp. 75-79

Spencer, E.Y. (1973) Guide to the Chemicals Used in Crop Protection, 6th ed., London, Ontario, University of Western Ontario, Research Branch, Agriculture Canada, Publication 1093

Stecher, P.G., ed. (1968) The Merck Index, 8th ed., Rahway, NJ, Merck & Co., p. 1047

US Code of Federal Regulations (1975) Air Contaminants, Title 29, part. 1910.1000, Washington DC, US Government Printing Office, p. 61

US Environmental Protection Agency (1974) EPA Compendium of Registered Pesticides, Vol. II, Fungicides and Nematicides, Washington DC, US Government Printing Office, pp. I-T-30-00.01-I-T-30-00.09

US International Trade Commission (1975a) Synthetic Organic Chemicals, US Production and Sales, 1973, ITC Publication 728, Washington DC, US Government Printing Office, pp. 137, 141

US International Trade Commission (1975b) Synthetic Organic Chemicals, US Production and Sales of Rubber-Processing Chemicals, 1974 Preliminary, Washington DC, US Government Printing Office, pp. 4, 8

US Tariff Commission (1926) Census of Dyes and Other Synthetic Organic Chemicals, 1925, Tariff Information Series No. 34, Washington DC, US Government Printing Office, p. 148

US Tariff Commision (1961) Synthetic Organic Chemicals, US Production and Sales, 1960, TC Publication 34, Washington DC, US Government Printing Office, p. 43

Weast, R.C., ed. (1975) CRC Handbook of Chemistry and Physics, 56th ed., Cleveland, Ohio, Chemical Rubber Co., p. C-272

Wenyon, C.E. (1972) Organic sulfur compounds. In: Chemical Technology: An Encyclopedic Treatment, Vol. 4, Petroleum and Organic Chemicals, New York, Barnes & Noble, pp. 621-623

WHO (1965) Evaluation of the toxicity of pesticide residues in food. WHO/Food Add./27.65, pp. 181-184

WHO (1975a) Pesticide residues in food. Report of the 1974 Joint Meeting of the FAO Working Party of Experts on Pesticide Residues and the WHO Expert Committee on Pesticide Residues. Wld Hlth Org. techn. Rep. Ser., No. 574, pp. 26-30

WHO (1975b) 1974 Evaluations of some pesticide residues in food. Wld Hlth Org. Pest. Res. Ser., No. 4, pp. 537-545

Winell, M.A. (1975) An international comparison of hygienic standards for chemicals in the work environment. Ambio, 4, 34-36

1. Chemical and Physical Data

1.1 Synonyms and trade names

Chem. Abstr. Reg. Serial No.: 315-18-4

Chem. Abstr. Name: 4-(Dimethylamino)-3,5-dimethylphenol methyl-carbamate (ester)

4-(Dimethylamino)-3,5-dimethylphenol, methylcarbamate; 4-dimethyl-amino-3,5-dimethylphenyl *N*-methylcarbamate; 4-(dimethylamino)-3,5-xylenol, methylcarbamate (ester); 4-dimethylamino-3,5-xylyl methyl-carbamate; 4-dimethylamino-3,5-xylyl *N*-methylcarbamate; methyl-carbamic acid, 4-(dimethylamino)-3,5-xylyl ester; methyl-4-dimethyl-amino-3,5-xylyl carbamate; methyl-4-dimethylamino-3,5-xylyl ester of carbamic acid

Dowco 139; ENT 25,766; Mexacarbate; Mexicarbate; Zactran; Zectane; Zextran

1.2 Chemical formula and molecular weight

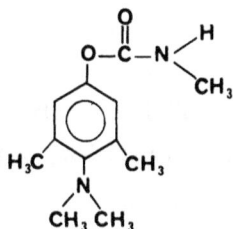

$C_{12}H_{18}N_2O_2$ Mol. wt: 222.3

1.3 Chemical and physical properties of the substance

From Stecher (1968), unless otherwise specified

(a) Description: Crystals

(b) Melting-point: 85°C

(c) Solubility: 0.01% soluble in water at 25°C; soluble in acetone, acetonitrile, ethanol, benzene and methylene chloride

(d) Volatility: Vapour pressure is <0.1 mm at 139°C.

(e) Stability: Hydrolyses rapidly in alkaline solution; subject to photo-decomposition in the solid state (Hosler, 1974)

1.4 Technical products and impurities

Zectran is no longer produced in the US but was formerly available as an emulsifiable concentrate containing 22.3% of the pure chemical, as a wettable powder containing 25% of the compound and as a bait formulation (Spencer, 1973).

2. Production, Use, Occurrence and Analysis

For important background information on this section, see preamble, p. 15.

2.1 Production and use

Zectran can be prepared by reductive alkylation of 4-nitroso-3,5-xylenol, followed by reaction with methyl isocyanate (Shulgin, 1962; Spencer, 1973).

It was produced on a pilot plant scale by one US company from 1961 until 1974 (Anon., 1975; Berg, 1976), but there is no evidence that the quantity produced exceeded a few thousand kg annually.

It is registered in the US for use as an insecticide and as a molluscicide for the control of many pests of lawns, turf and flowers (US Environmental Protection Agency, 1974) but not for use on food crops. In 1975, 15 thousand kg were applied in an emergency measure to control an outbreak of spruce budworm in the state of Maine (Anon., 1975).

2.2 Occurrence

Zectran is not known to occur as a natural product.

2.3 Analysis

A general method for the analysis of organic pollutants in water and waste water has been applied to zectran (Lichtenberg, 1975). Chromatographic methods for the analysis of carbamates, including zectran, have been reviewed (Fishbein & Zielinski, 1967; Sherma, 1973).

Gas chromatography and a nitrogen- or sulphur-responsive alkali flame detector were used to analyse plant extracts for zectran (Lorah & Hemphill, 1974). Electron-capture gas chromatography has been used after derivatization with pentafluoropropionic anhydride (Sherma & Shafik, 1975). Zectran was separated from several other pesticides by thin-layer chromatography; the limit of sensitivity was 0.2 µg (Ebing, 1972). A method involving fluorigenic labelling, thin-layer chromatography and *in situ* fluorimetry is capable of detecting 15 ng zectran on a routine basis; the limit of detection was 1 ng (Frei & Lawrence, 1972).

A water monitoring system for cholinesterase inhibitors, including, but not specific for, zectran, uses an electrochemical cell which measures changes in the activity of immobilized enzymes (Goodson & Jacobs, 1972).

3. Biological Data Relevant to the Evaluation of Carcinogenic Risk to Man

3.1 Carcinogenicity and related studies in animals

(a) Oral administration

Mouse: Groups of 18 male and 18 female (C57BL/6xC3H/Anf)F_1 mice and 18 male and 18 female (C57BL/6xAKR)F_1 mice received commercial zectran (95% pure) according to the following schedule: 4.64 mg/kg bw in gelatine at 7 days of age by stomach tube and the same amount (not adjusted for increasing body weight) daily up to 4 weeks of age; subsequently, the mice were given 11 mg zectran per kg of diet. The dose was the maximum tolerated dose for infant and young mice but not necessarily so for adults. The experiment was terminated when the animals were about 78 weeks of age, at which time 14, 17, 17 and 16 mice in the four groups, respectively, were still alive. Tumour incidences were compared with those observed among 79-90 necropsied mice of each sex and strain, which either had been untreated or had received gelatine only: the incidences were increased in males of the first strain (9/16 *versus* 22/79) [P<0.05] but not in females of the same strain nor in either sex of the second strain. The incidence of lung adenomas was increased in both sexes of the first strain (4/16 in males and 3/17 in females *versus* 5/79 and 3/87 controls ; if both sexes are considered together, P<0.01). Hepatomas were found in 5/16 males of the first strain, compared with 8/79 in controls [P<0.05], and in 2/17 males of the second strain, compared with 5/90 in controls [P>0.05]. No hepatomas were seen in females (Innes *et al.*, 1969; NTIS, 1968).

(b) Subcutaneous administration

Mouse: Groups of 18 male and 18 female (C57BL/6xC3H/Anf)F_1 mice and 18 male and 18 female (C57BL/6xAKR)F_1 mice were given single s.c. injections of 10 mg/kg bw commercial zectran (95% pure) in dimethyl sulphoxide on the 28th day of life and were observed until they were about 78 weeks of age, at which time 17, 18, 17 and 17 mice in the four groups, respectively, were still alive. Tumour incidences were compared with those in groups of 141, 154, 161 and 157 untreated or vehicle-injected controls that were necropsied. Incidences were not increased (P>0.05) for any tumour type in any sex-strain subgroup or in the combined sexes of either strain (NTIS, 1968) [The Working Group noted that a negative result obtained with a single s.c. injection may not be an adequate basis for discounting carcinogenicity].

3.2 Other relevant biological data

(a) Experimental systems

The oral and dermal LD_{50}'s of zectran in rats are 14-63 and 1500-2500 mg/kg bw, respectively (Ben-Dyke *et al.*, 1970). A single percutaneous application of 2000 mg/kg bw produced no discernible effects in New Zealand rabbits (Tucker & Crabtree, 1969). Zectran inhibits acetylcholinesterase activity (Kuhr & Dorough, 1976).

Meikle (1973) has provided a concise review of zectran metabolism. In dogs, an oral dose of zectran was eliminated quantitatively in the urine as 4-dimethylamino-3,5-xylenol, predominantly in the conjugated form, as conjugated forms of the 2,6-dimethyl hydroquinone, and as small amounts of 2,6-

dimethyl-*para*-benzoquinone (Williams *et al.*, 1964).

Dog and rat liver homogenates, dog kidney homogenates (Wheeler & Strother, 1971) and rat-liver microsomes (Oonnithan & Casida, 1966) metabolized zectran into a mixture of metabolites, including 4-dimethylamino-3,5-xylyl-*N*-hydroxy-methylcarbamate, 4-methylformamido-3,5-xylyl methylcarbamate, 4-methylamino-3,5-xylyl methylcarbamate and 4-amino-3,5-xylyl methylcarbamate. 4-Dimethyl-amino-3,5-xylyl-*N*-hydroxymethylcarbamate was formed (6%) in a rat-liver preparation but not in a human-liver preparation (Bedford, 1975).

It caused an increase in the number of reverse mutations in *Bacillus subtilis* (De Giovanni-Donnelly *et al.*, 1968); metabolic activation was not used in this test.

(b) Man

In an incident of acute zectran poisoning, the blood acetylcholine-sterase level was lowered but returned to normal after 3 days (Richardson & Batteese, 1973).

3.3 Case reports and epidemiological studies

No data were available to the Working Group.

4. Comments on Data Reported and Evaluation

4.1 Animal data

Zectran has been tested by oral administration and by single subcutaneous injection in two strains of mice. Following its oral admini-stration, an increased incidence of lung adenomas was observed in both sexes of one strain combined, together with a slight increase in the number of liver-cell tumours in males of the same strain. The available data do not allow an evaluation of the carcinogenicity of zectran to be made.

4.2 Human data

No case reports or epidemiological studies were available to the Working Group.

5. References

Anon. (1975) Forest pests pestered. Chemical Week, June 25, p. 18

Bedford, C. (1975) Biotransformations: agricultural and industrial chemicals. In: Hathway, D.E., ed., Foreign Compound Metabolism in Mammals, London, The Chemical Society

Ben-Dyke, R., Sanderson, D.M. & Noakes, D.N. (1970) Acute toxicity data for pesticides. Wld Rev. Pest. Control, 9, 119-127

Berg, G.L., ed. (1976) Farm Chemicals Handbook 1975, Willoughby, Ohio, Meister, p. D 273

De Giovanni-Donnelly, R., Kolbye, S.M. & Greeves, P.D. (1968) The effects of IPC, CIPC, sevin and zectran on *Bacillus subtilis*. Experientia, 24, 80-81

Ebing, W. (1972) Routinemethode zur Dünnschichtchromatographischen Identifizierung der Pestizidrückstände aus den Klassen der Triazine, Carbamate, Harnstoffe und Uracile. J. Chromat., 65, 533-545

Fishbein, L. & Zielinski, W.L., Jr, (1967) Chromatography of carbamates. Chromat. Rev., 9, 37-101

Frei, R.W. & Lawrence, J.F. (1972) Determination of matacil and zectran by fluorigenic labeling, thin layer chromatography, and *in situ* fluorimetry. J. Ass. off. analyt. Chem., 55, 1259-1264

Goodson, L.H. & Jacobs, W.B. (1972) Rapid Detection System for Organophosphates and Carbamate Insecticides in Water, EPA-R2-72-010, Washington DC, US Environmental Protection Agency

Hosler, C.F., Jr (1974) Degradation of zectran in alkaline water. Bull. environm. Contam. Toxicol., 12, 599-605

Innes, J.R.M., Ulland, B.M., Valerio, M.G., Petrucelli, L., Fishbein, L., Hart, E.R., Pallotta, A.J., Bates, R.R., Falk, H.L., Gart, J.J., Klein, M., Mitchell, I. & Peters, J. (1969) Bioassay of pesticides and industrial chemicals for tumorigenicity in mice: a preliminary note. J. nat. Cancer Inst., 42, 1101-1114

Kuhr, R.J. & Dorough, H.W. (1976) Carbamate Insecticides: Chemistry, Biochemistry and Toxicology, Cleveland, Ohio, Chemical Rubber Co., pp. 44-47

Lichtenberg, J.J. (1975) Methods for the determination of specific organic pollutants in water and waste water. Inst. Electrical Electronics Engineers Trans. Nuclear Sci., NS-22, 874-891

Lorah, E.J. & Hemphill, D.D. (1974) Direct chromatography of some *N*-methyl-carbamate pesticides. J. Ass. off. analyt. Chem., 57, 570-575

Meikle, R.W. (1973) Metabolism of 4-dimethylamino-3,5-xylyl methylcarbamate (mexacarbamate, active ingredient of zectran insecticide): a unified picture. Bull. environm. Contam. Toxicol., 10, 29-36

NTIS (National Technical Information Service) (1968) Evaluation of Carcino-genic, Teratogenic and Mutagenic Activities of Selected Pesticides and Industrial Chemicals, Vol. 1, Carcinogenic Study, Washington DC, US Department of Commerce

Oonnithan, E.S. & Casida, J.E. (1966) Metabolites of methyl- and dimethyl-carbamate insecticide chemicals as formed by rat liver microsomes. Bull. environm. Contam. Toxicol., 1, 59-69

Richardson, E.M. & Batteese, R.I., Jr (1973) An incident of zectran poison-ing. J. Maine med. Ass., 64, 158-159

Sherma, J. (1973) Chromatographic analysis of pesticide residues. CRC Crit. Rev. analyt. Chem., 3, 299-354

Sherma, J. & Shafik, T.M. (1975) A multiclass, multiresidue analytical method for determining pesticide residues in air. Arch. environm. Contam. Toxicol., 3, 55-71

Shulgin, A.T. (1962) *p*-Aminophenyl carbamates. US Patent 3,060,225, October 23, to Dow Chemical Co.

Spencer, E.Y. (1973) Guide to the Chemicals Used in Crop Protection, 6th ed., London, Ontario, University of Western Ontario, Research Branch, Agriculture Canada, Publication 1093, p. 354

Stecher, P.G., ed. (1968) The Merck Index, 8th ed., Rahway, NJ, Merck & Co., pp. 1126-1127

Tucker, R.K. & Crabtree, D.G. (1969) Toxicity of zectran insecticide to several wildlife species. J. econ. Entomol., 62, 1307-1310

US Environmental Protection Agency (1974) EPA Compendium of Registered Pesticides, Washington DC, US Government Printing Office, p. III-D-37.1

Wheeler, L. & Strother, A. (1971) *In vitro* metabolism of the *N*-methylcar-bamates, zectran and mesurol, by liver, kidney and blood of dogs and rats. J. Pharmacol. exp. Ther., 178, 371-382

Williams, E., Meikle, R.W. & Redemann, C.T. (1964) Identification of meta-bolites of zectran insecticide in dog urine. J. agric. Fd Chem., 12, 457-461

ZINEB

1. Chemical and Physical Data

1.1 Synonyms and trade names

Chem. Abstr. Reg. Serial No.: 12122-67-7

Chem. Abstr. Name: {[1,2-Ethanediylbis(carbamodithioato)] (2-)}zinc

{[1,2-Ethanediylbis(carbamodithioato)] (2-)}-*S*,*S*'-zinc; 1,2-ethanediylbiscarbamodithioic acid, zinc complex; 1,2-ethane-diylbiscarbamothioic acid, zinc salt; [ethylenebis(dithiocarbamate)]-zinc; ethylenebis(dithiocarbamato)zinc; zinc ethylene bisdithio-carbamate

Aspor; Asporum; Bercema; Blizene; Carbadine; Chem Zineb; Cineb; Crittox; Cynkotox; Daisen; Dithane 65; Dithane Z; Dithane Z 78; Hexathane; Kupratsin; Kypzin; Lirotan; Lonacol; Micide; Miltox; Novosir N; Novozin N 50; Novozir; Novozir N; Novozir N 50; Pamosol 2 Forte; Parzate; Parzate C; Parzate zineb; Perosin; Perosin 75B; Perozin; Perozine; Polyram Z; Tiezene; Tritoftorol; Zebenide; Zebtox; Zidan; Zineb 80; Zinosan

1.2 Chemical formula and molecular weight

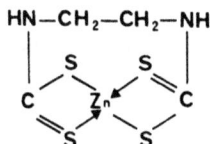

$$HN-CH_2-CH_2-NH$$

$C_4H_6N_2S_4Zn$ Mol. wt: 275.8

1.3 Chemical and physical properties of the substance

From Stecher (1968), unless otherwise specified

(a) Description: Powder or crystals

(b) Solubility: Insoluble in water at room temperature; soluble in chloroform, carbon disulphide and pyridine

(c) Stability: Decomposes before melting (Spencer, 1973)

1.4 Technical products and impurities

Zineb is available in the US as dusts containing 3.25-19.5% of the chemical, as wettable powders containing 1.4 to 75% of the chemical and as a 39% aqueous suspension (US Environmental Protection Agency, 1974). Technical zineb is available in Japan in grades containing 90%, 93% or 95% of the chemical (Japanese Ministry of Agriculture & Forestry, 1975).

Many commercial samples of ethylenebisdithiocarbamates, including zineb, have been shown to contain ethylenethiourea (ETU) (Bontoyan *et al.*, 1972). Bontoyan & Looker (1973) studied the initial ETU contents of various such products and the levels found after storage at $88^{\circ}C$. The initial content in specific formulations of 'Zineb 80%' varied between 0.16 and 2%; after 39 days of storage the levels were between 3.5 and 10.5%.

2. Production, Use, Occurrence and Analysis

For important background information on this section, see preamble, p. 15.

2.1 Production and use

Zineb is believed to have been first prepared in 1941 (Hester, 1943). The method thought to be used for its commercial production is reaction of ethylene diamine with carbon disulphide in the presence of alkali, followed by addition of zinc sulphate to precipitate zineb. This final step can also be carried out in a spray tank by the so-called 'tank-mix' of sodium or ammonium ethylenebisdithiocarbamate with zinc sulphate (US Environmental Protection Agency, 1974).

Since only two companies currently produce zineb in the US, separate production data are not available; however, in 1974 production of a group of at least 9 dithiocarbamate fungicides, including zineb, was 16 million kg (US International Trade Commission, 1975). The highest reported production of zineb in the US was 3.8 million kg in 1961; 1.4 million kg were produced in 1968, the last year in which production was reported separately.

Most of the 1.7 million kg of sodium ethylenebisdithiocarbamate produced in 1961 and the 0.9 million kg made in 1968 was probably converted to zineb by the tank-mix procedure (US Tariff Commission, 1962, 1969). Total US exports of all dithiocarbamates, including zineb, in 1974 were 6.7 million kg (US Department of Agriculture, 1975).

It is estimated that the annual production of zineb in Italy is 10-20 million kg, 5 million kg of which is used within the country. Annual production in Spain is 1-5 million kg and that in France, less than 1 million kg. It is also produced in the Federal Republic of Germany and The Netherlands (Berg, 1976).

Production of zineb in Japan began in 1952; two companies produced 2 million kg in 1974. In that year, 235 thousand kg of formulated zineb were imported into Japan from France, Israel and the US. In earlier years, minor quantities of zineb formulations were exported from Japan to countries in south-east Asia, but none were reported in 1973 or 1974 (Japanese Ministry of Agriculture & Forestry, 1975).

Zineb is a fungicide and is registered for use in the US on over 50 fruit, vegetable and field crops, as well as on a large number of ornamental plants and for the treatment of many seeds. Residue tolerances are established at 7 mg/kg for most raw agricultural crop products. Zineb is also registered for use as a fungicide in paints and for mould control on fabrics, leather, linen, painted surfaces, surfaces to be painted and paper, plastic and wood surfaces (US Environmental Protection Agency, 1974).

In Japan, over half of the 1.8 million kg used in 1974 was on citrus fruits; most of the balance was used on vegetables, and a small amount was used on flowers (Japanese Ministry of Agriculture & Forestry, 1975).

In December 1974, the Joint Meeting of the FAO Working Party of Experts on Pesticide Residues and the WHO Expert Committee on Pesticide Residues established a revised temporary acceptable daily intake for man of 0-0.005 mg/kg bw for all dithiocarbamate fungicides (WHO, 1975a,b).

2.2 Occurrence

Zineb is not known to occur as a natural product.

As part of the 'Total Diet Program' of the US Food and Drug Administration, 360 composite food samples were collected annually during the
period 1964-1970, prepared as for consumption and analysed for dithiocarbamate content. A maximum of 4 composites contained detectable levels
of dithiocarbamates in any single year (Corneliussen, 1972), and in at
least one year no dithiocarbamate was detected. On the basis of these
results, analysis for dithiocarbamates in this programme was discontinued
after 1970 (Manske & Corneliussen, 1974).

The significance of zineb as a residue on agricultural products is
enhanced by reports that the cooking of foods containing ethylenebisdithiocarbamate residues would result in degradation to form ETU. Studies
indicate that normal cooking of vegetables containing residues of zineb
near the tolerance level would result in the formation and possible human
consumption of ETU (Blasquez, 1973; Watts *et al.*, 1974). For information
on the levels of ETU that may be found on raw agricultural products, see
IARC (1974).

2.3 Analysis

Two reviews have described methods of analysis for zineb (Fishbein,
1975; Fishbein & Zielinski, 1967). Gas chromatography has been used to
determine zineb in food and feeds (Bighi, 1964); another gas chromatographic method depends on the analysis of ethylenediamine, which is formed
as a hydrolysis product of ethylenebisdithiocarbamate pesticides (Newsome,
1974).

Stevenson (1972) has described a test based on the colour developed
by acid dithizone, which depends on the type and concentration of metal
present. However, the presence of a dithiocarbamate must be established
separately, using conventional procedures. Polarographic methods have
also been used (Budnikov *et al.*, 1974; Supin *et al.*, 1973).

3. Biological Data Relevant to the Evaluation
of Carcinogenic Risk to Man

3.1 Carcinogenicity and related studies in animals

(a) Oral administration

Mouse: Groups of 18 male and 18 female (C57BL/6xC3H/Anf)F_1 mice and
18 male and 18 female (C57BL/6xAKR)F_1 mice received commercial zineb (97%
pure) according to the following schedule: 464 mg/kg bw in gelatine at
7 days of age by stomach tube and the same amount (not adjusted for
increasing body weight) daily up to 4 weeks of age; subsequently, the
mice were given 1298 mg zineb per kg of diet. The dose given was the
maximum tolerated dose for infant and young mice but not necessarily so
for adults. The experiment was terminated when the animals were about
78 weeks of age, at which time 15, 18, 16 and 16 mice in the four groups,
respectively, were still alive. Tumour incidences were compared with
those observed among 79-90 necropsied mice of each sex and strain, which
either had been untreated or had received gelatine only: the incidences
were not significantly greater (P>0.05) for any tumour type in any sex-
strain subgroup or in the combined sexes of either strain (Innes *et al.*,
1969; NTIS, 1968).

Of 101 strain A mice and 79 C57BL mice given weekly oral doses of
3500 mg/kg bw zineb (purity unspecified) in 1% starch solution for 6 weeks
and killed 3 months after the beginning of the experiment, 35/101 (35%)
and 6/79 (8%) developed lung adenomas. Among controls, 30/97 (31%) strain
A mice and 0/87 C57BL mice developed lung adenomas [for C57BL mice, P=0.01].
Of 29 C57BL mice given 11 weekly doses of 1750 mg/kg bw by stomach tube
and killed 6 months after the beginning of the experiment, 2 (7%) developed
lung adenomas, compared with 0/59 controls (Chernov & Khitsenko, 1969).

Rat: A group of 60 random-bred rats was given twice weekly doses of
285 mg/kg bw commercial zineb (89.6% pure) in water by stomach tube for up
to 22 months, at which time 10 survived; 2 had tumours (1 adenocarcinoma
and 1 lymphosarcoma of the intestine). One of 46 untreated controls still
alive at 22 months developed a fibrosarcoma (Andrianova & Alekseev, 1970)
[P>0.05].

Groups of 10 rats of each sex were given 0 (control), 500, 1000, 2500, 5000 or 10,000 mg zineb (purity unspecified) per kg of diet for 2 years. Of 15 animals which died within 1 year, 8 were among those fed the two highest dose levels. Among male animals, there was 1 tumour-bearing animal in the controls, 2 fed 500 mg/kg, 3 fed 1000 mg/kg, 2 fed 2500 mg/kg, 1 fed 5000 mg/kg and 1 fed 10,000 mg/kg. Among females, the corresponding figures were 1, 0, 1, 1, 0 and 0. The tumours were malignant tumours of the lung, with the exception of an additional malignant tumour in the small bowel of 1 male fed 10,000 mg/kg, a mammary carcinoma in 1 female fed 1000 mg/kg and a papillary adenocarcinoma of the thyroid in 1 female fed 2500 mg/kg (Blackwell-Smith *et al.*, 1953).

(b) Subcutaneous administration

Mouse: Groups of 18 male and 18 female (C57BL/6xC3H/Anf)F_1 mice and 18 male and 18 female (C57BL/6xAKR)F_1 mice were given single s.c. injections of 1000 mg/kg bw commercial zineb (97% pure) in 0.5% gelatine at 28 days of age and were observed until they were about 78 weeks of age, at which time 16, 18, 18 and 17 mice in the four groups, respectively, were still alive. Tumour incidences were compared with **those** in groups of 141, 154, 161 and 157 untreated or vehicle-injected controls that were necropsied. In males of the first strain, 5/18 autopsied mice had developed systemic reticulum-cell sarcomas, compared with 8/141 controls [P<0.01]. There was no other increase in tumour incidence over that in controls (NTIS, 1968).

Rat: A group of 48 non-inbred rats received 20 mg/kg bw commercial zineb (89.6% pure) as a s.c. implant in a 250 mg paraffin pellet. Of the 6 rats still alive at 22 months, 4 developed tumours (1 malignant hepatoma, 1 fibrosarcoma, 1 spindle-cell sarcoma and 1 rhabdomyosarcoma). One of 46 untreated controls, which did not received paraffin pellets and were still alive at 22 months, developed a fibrosarcoma (Andrianova & Alekseev, 1970) [P<0.001].

(c) Other experimental systems

Prenatal exposure: Of 18 pregnant female A mice that received single i.p. injections of 8 mg/animal zineb (purity unspecified) during the second half of pregnancy, 11 produced a total of 38 offspring, 20 of which survived.

These were killed and examined at the age of 4 months, and lung adenomas were found in 6. Lung adenomas had not been observed in 4-month old mice of that strain in the same laboratory (Kvitnitskaya & Kolesnichenko, 1971).

3.2 Other relevant biological data

(a) Experimental systems

The oral LD_{50} of zineb in rats is 1-8 g/kg bw (Ben-Dyke et al., 1970; Blackwell-Smith et al., 1953). Groups of 4-week old rats were given 500-10,000 mg zineb per kg of diet for 2 years; there was some mortality among females fed 5000 and 10,000 mg/kg, and a goitrogenic effect was observed at all dose levels. Hyperplasia of the thyroid was seen in dogs given up to 10,000 mg zineb per kg of diet for 1 year (Blackwell-Smith et al., 1953).

In rats, the breakdown of zineb (1) (Scheme 1) into ethylene diamine (2) and carbon disulphide may occur under the acid conditions of the stomach. This would account for part of the carbon disulphide that is excreted in the exhaled air (Truhaut et al., 1973); the remainder arises from the transformation of ethylene bisthiuram monosulphide (3) into ETU (4) (Engst et al., 1971). The absorbed ethylene diamine (2) is partly eliminated via the lungs as carbon dioxide and the remainder in ionized form in the urine. 'Ethylene bis-isothiocyanate', for which two alternative structures (5 and 6) are proposed*, possibly ethylene bisthiuram monosulphide (3) and another unidentified zineb metabolite are also detected in the urine (Truhaut et al., 1973).

When rats were dosed with 100 mg/kg bw/day for periods of up to 6 months, first pregnancies were retarded, and there was an increased incidence of sterility and foetal resorption. The resulting neonates had crooked tails and suffered most noticeably from a reduced or retarded weight gain; there were some early postnatal deaths. Toxic effects also occurred

---

*The Working Group considered the probable structure to be that represented in (6).

SCHEME 1

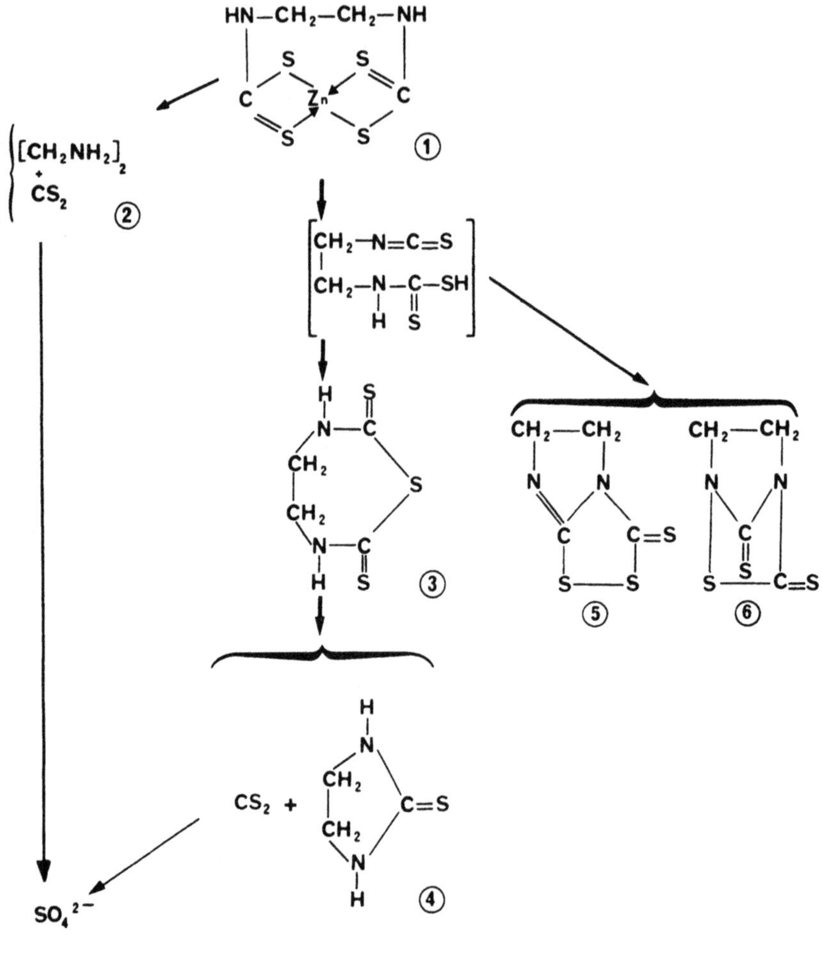
HN—CH2—CH2—NH
S
S
C
Zn
C
S
S
①
[CH2NH2]2
+
CS2
②
CH2—N=C=S
CH2—N—C—SH
H
S
H
S
N—C
CH2
S
CH2
N—C
H
S
③
CH2—CH2
N
N
C
C=S
S—S
⑤
CH2—CH2
N
N
C
S
S—C=S
⑥
H
N
CH2
C=S
CH2
N
H
④
CS2 +
SO4 2−

in those neonates that continued to receive zineb at the same dose level as their parents (Ryazanova, 1967).

Single oral doses of 2-8 g/kg bw administered to pregnant rats on day 11 or 13 of pregnancy resulted in congenital abnormalities in 12-100% of the foetuses. The maximum dose level at which no teratogenic effect was observed was 1 g/kg bw: no adverse effect on the intra-uterine development of the progeny was observed when this dose was given daily to groups of rats from day 2 to day 21 of pregnancy, or when the rats were exposed by inhalation to a concentration of 100 mg zineb/m^3 for 4 hours per day from day 4 of pregnancy (Petrova-Vergieva & Ivanova-Chemishanska, 1971, 1973).

(b) Man

One person suffering from hypocatalasaemia developed sulphaemoglobinaemia, haemolytic anaemia and Heinz body formation after contact with zineb (Pinkhas *et al.*, 1963). An increase in the number of chromosome aberrations in peripheral blood lymphocytes was observed in a study of persons occupationally exposed to zineb (Pilinskaya, 1974).

(c) Carcinogenicity of metabolites

ETU (4) (Scheme 1) produced thyroid carcinomas in rats and increased the incidence of liver-cell tumours in two strains of mice after its oral administration (IARC, 1974).

3.3 Case reports and epidemiological studies

No data were available to the Working Group.

4. Comments on Data Reported and Evaluation

4.1 Animal data

Zineb produced an increased incidence of lung tumours after its oral administration to mice of one strain. Systemic reticulum-cell sarcomas were observed in mice and a variety of sarcomas in rats after its subcutaneous administration. No increases in tumour incidences were observed in two other strains of mice and in two limited studies in rats following oral administration. The available data do not allow an evaluation of the

253

carcinogenicity of zineb to be made.

4.2 Human data

No case reports or epidemiological studies were available to the Working Group.

5. References

Andrianova, M.M. & Alekseev, I.V. (1970) On the carcinogenic properties of the pesticides sevine, maneb, ciram and cineb. Vop. Pitan., 29, 71-74

Ben-Dyke, R., Sanderson, D.M. & Noakes, D.N. (1970) Acute toxicity data for pesticides. Wld Rev. Pest. Control, 9, 119-127

Berg, G.L., ed. (1976) Farm Chemicals Handbook 1975, Willoughby, Ohio, Meister, p. D 222

Bighi, C. (1964) Microdetermination of dithiocarbamates by gas chromatography. J. Chromat., 14, 348-354

Blackwell-Smith, R., Jr, Finnegan, J.K., Larson, P.S., Sahyoun, P.F., Dreyfuss, M.L. & Haag, H.B. (1953) Toxicologic studies on zinc and disodium ethylene bisdithiocarbamates. J. Pharmacol. exp. Ther., 109, 159-166

Blasquez, C.H. (1973) Residue determination of ethylenethiourea (2-imidazolidinethione) from tomato foliage, soil and water. J. agric. Fd Chem., 21, 330-332

Bontoyan, W.R. & Looker, J.B. (1973) Degradation of commercial ethylene bisdithiocarbamate formulations to ethylenethiourea under elevated temperature and humidity. J. agric. Fd Chem., 21, 338-342

Bontoyan, W.R., Looker, J.B., Kaiser, T.E., Giang, P. & Olive, B.M. (1972) Survey of ethylenethiourea in commercial ethylenebisdithiocarbamate formulations. J. Ass. off. analyt. Chem., 55, 923-925

Budnikov, G.K., Toropova, V.F., Ulakhovich, N.A. & Viter, I.P. (1974) Electrochemical behavior of dithiocarbamates on a mercury electrode. III. Polarographic study of fungicides of dithiocarbamate type in organic solvents. Zh. analyt. Khim., 29, 1204-1209

Chernov, O.V. & Khitsenko, I.I. (1969) Blastomogenic properties of some derivatives of dithiocarbamic acid. Vop. Onkol., 15, 71-74

Corneliussen, P.E. (1972) Pesticide residues in total diet samples. VI. Pest. Monit. J., 5, 313-330

Engst, R., Schnaak, W. & Lewerenz, H.-J. (1971) Untersuchungen zum Metabolismus der Fungiciden Äthylen-bis-dithiocarbamate Maneb, Zineb und Nabam. V. Zur Toxikologie der Abbauprodukte. Z. Lebensmitt.-Untersuch., 146, 91-97

Fishbein, L. (1975) Chromatography of Environmental Hazards, Vol. 3, Pesticides, Amsterdam, Elsevier, pp. 676-692

Fishbein, L. & Zielinski, W.L., Jr (1967) Chromatography of carbamates. Chromat. Rev., 9, 37-101

Hester, W.F. (1943) Fungicidal composition. US Patent 2,317,765, April 27, to Röhm & Haas Co.

IARC (1974) IARC Monographs on the Evaluation of Carcinogenic Risk of Chemicals to Man, 7, Some Anti-thyroid and Related Substances, Nitrofurans and Industrial Chemicals, Lyon, pp. 45-52

Innes, J.R.M., Ulland, B.M., Valerio, M.G., Petrucelli, L., Fishbein, L., Hart, E.R., Pallotta, A.J., Bates, R.R., Falk, H.L., Gart, J.J., Klein, M., Mitchell, I. & Peters, J. (1969) Bioassay of pesticides and industrial chemicals for tumorigenicity in mice: a preliminary note. J. nat. Cancer Inst., 42, 1101-1114

Japanese Ministry of Agriculture and Forestry (1975) Noyaku Yoran (Agricultural Chemicals Annual), 1975, Division of Plant Disease Prevention, Tokyo, Takeo Endo, pp. 17-19, 26, 89, 101, 265, 301

Kvitnitskaya, V.A. & Kolesnichenko, T.S. (1971) On the transplacental blastomogenous action of cineb on the progeny of mice. Vop. Pitan., 30, 49-50

Manske, D.D. & Corneliussen, P.E. (1974) Pesticide residues in total diet samples. VII. Pest. Monit. J., 8, 110-114

Newsome, W.H. (1974) A method for determining ethylenebis(dithiocarbamate) residues on food crops as bis(trifluoroacetamido)ethane. J. agric. Fd Chem., 22, 886-889

NTIS (National Technical Information Service) (1968) Evaluation of Carcinogenic, Teratogenic and Mutagenic Activities of Selected Pesticides and Industrial Chemicals, Vol. 1, Carcinogenic Study, Washington DC, US Department of Commerce

Petrova-Vergieva, T. & Ivanova-Chemishanska, L. (1971) On the teratogenic effect of zinc ethylenebisdithiocarbamate (zineb) in rats. Eksp. Med. Morfol., 10, 226-230

Petrova-Vergieva, T. & Ivanova-Chemishanska, L. (1973) Assessment of the teratogenic activity of dithiocarbamate fungicides. Fd Cosmet. Toxicol., 11, 239-244

Pilinskaya, M.A. (1974) Results of cytogenetic examination of persons occupationally contacting with the fungicide zineb. Genetika, 10, 140-146

Pinkhas, J., Djaldetti, M., Joshua, H., Resnick, C. & de Vries, A. (1963) Sulfhemoglobinemia and acute hemolytic anemia with Heinz bodies following contact with a fungicide - zinc ethylene bisdithiocarbamate - in a subject with glucose-6-phosphate dehydrogenase deficiency and hypocatalasemia. Blood, 21, 484-494

Ryazanova, R.A. (1967) Effect of the fungicides ciram and cineb on the generative function of test animals. Gig. i Sanit., 32, 26-30

Spencer, E.Y. (1973) Guide to the Chemicals Used in Crop Protection, 6th ed., London, Ontario, University of Western Ontario, Research Branch, Agriculture Canada, Publication 1093, p. 537

Stecher, P.G., ed. (1968) The Merck Index, 8th ed., Rahway, NJ, Merck & Co., p. 1131

Stevenson, A. (1972) A simple color spot test for distinguishing between maneb, zineb, mancozeb, and selected mixtures. J. Ass. off. analyt. Chem., 55, 939-941

Supin, G.S., Klisenko, M.A. & Vekshtein, M.S. (1973) Polarographic determination of residual amounts of fungicide as dithiocarbonic acid derivatives. Khim. selsk. Khozyaistve, 11, 840-842

Truhaut, R., Fujita, M., Lich, N.P. & Chaigneau, M. (1973) Etude des transformations métaboliques du zinèbe (éthylènebisdithiocarbamate de zinc) chez le rat. C.R. Acad. Sci. (Paris), 276, 229-233

US Department of Agriculture (1975) The Pesticide Review 1974, Washington DC, US Government Printing Office, p. 11

US Environmental Protection Agency (1974) EPA Compendium of Registered Pesticides, Vol. 2, Washington DC, US Government Printing Office, pp. Z-10-00.01 - Z-10-00.17

US International Trade Commission (1975) Synthetic Organic Chemicals, US Production and Sales of Pesticides and Related Products, 1974 Preliminary, US Government Printing Office, Washington DC, p. 3

US Tariff Commission (1962) Synthetic Organic Chemicals, US Production and Sales, 1961, TC Publication 72, US Government Printing Office, Washington DC, p. 50

US Tariff Commission (1969) Synthetic Organic Chemicals, US Production and Sales, 1968, TC Publication 327, US Government Printing Office, Washington DC, p. 199

Watts, R.R., Storherr, R.W. & Onley, J.H. (1974) Effects of cooking on ethylenebisdithiocarbamate degradation to ethylene thiourea. Bull. environm. Contam. Toxicol., 12, 224-226

WHO (1975a) 1974 Evaluations of some pesticide residues in food. Wld Hlth Org. Pest. Res. Ser., No. 4, pp. 261-262

WHO (1975b) Pesticide residues in food. Report of the 1974 Joint Meeting of the FAO Working Party of Experts on Pesticide Residues and the WHO Expert Committee on Pesticide Residues. Wld Hlth Org. techn. Rep. Ser., No. 574, pp. 26-30

ZIRAM

1. Chemical and Physical Data

1.1 Synonyms and trade names

Chem. Abstr. Reg. Serial No.: 137-30-4

Chem. Abstr. Name: Bis(dimethylcarbamodithioato-S,S')zinc

Bis(dimethyldithiocarbamato)zinc; dimethylcarbamodithioic acid, zinc complex; dimethylcarbamodithioic acid, zinc salt; dimethyl-dithiocarbamate zinc salt; dimethyldithiocarbamic acid, zinc salt; methyl zimate; methyl ziram; zinc bis(dimethyldithiocarbamate); zinc bis(dimethyldithiocarbamoyl)disulphide; zinc dimethyl dithio-carbamate; zinc N-dimethyldithiocarbamate; zinc N,N-dimethyldithio-carbamate

Accelerator L; Aceto ZDED; Aceto ZDMD; Alcobam ZM; Carbazinc; Corona Corozate; Corozate; Cuman; Cymate; Eptac 1; Fuclasin; Fuklasin; Hexazir; Karbam White; Methasan; Methazate; Mezene; Milbam; Milban; Molurame; Orchard brand Ziram; Pomarzol Z-forte; Rhodiacid; Soxinal PZ; Soxinol PZ; Tricarbamix Z; Triscabol; Vancide MZ-96; Vulcacure ZM; Vulkacit L; Vulkacite L; Z 75; Z-C Spray; Zerlate; Zimate; Zirame; Zirberk; Ziride; Zitox

1.2 Chemical formula and molecular weight

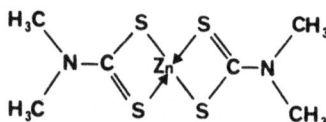

$C_6H_{12}N_2S_4Zn$ Mol. wt: 305.8

1.3 Chemical and physical properties of the substance

From Stecher (1968), unless otherwise specified

(a) Description: White powder or crystals

(b) Melting-point: $250^{\circ}C$ (crystals); $148^{\circ}C$ (dust)

(c) Solubility: Insoluble in water; slightly soluble in carbon tetrachloride, diethyl ether and ethanol (0.2 g/100 ml at $25^{\circ}C$); 0.5 g or less are soluble in 100 ml of acetone, benzene and other non-polar solvents.

1.4 Technical products and impurities

Ziram is available in the US as dusts containing 3.5-76% of the chemical, as wettable powders containing 30-96% of the chemical, as aqueous suspensions containing 30-40% of the chemical and as a 0.1% paste (US Environmental Protection Agency, 1973).

In Japan, ziram is available as a technical grade product containing 98% of the chemical and less than 0.5% water, 0.4-0.5% sodium chloride and 1.0-1.1% other impurities (mostly zinc methyldithiocarbamate) (Japanese Ministry of Agriculture & Forestry, 1975).

2. Production, Use, Occurrence and Analysis

For important background information on this section, see preamble, p. 15.

2.1 Production and use

Ziram can be prepared from zinc oxide, dimethylamine and carbon disulphide (Stecher, 1968). It was first produced commercially in the US as a fungicide in 1947 (US Tariff Commission, 1949) but had been used as a rubber accelerator since 1943 (US Tariff Commission, 1945). In 1973, ziram was produced in the US by eight companies whose combined production amounted to 1 million kg.

It is estimated to be produced in Italy at a rate of 1-5 million kg annually, and in the Benelux countries, the Federal Republic of Germany,

France, Spain and the UK in amounts of less than 1 million kg annually in each country.

Ziram was first produced in Japan in 1969; approximately 2.7 thousand kg were produced in 1970 and about 700 kg in 1973. Two Japanese companies are currently producing this chemical (Japanese Ministry of Agriculture & Forestry, 1975).

The usefulness of ziram as a fungicide was first observed in 1944 (McCallan, 1967). It is registered in the US for use on 24 fruit and vegetable crops and on several commercial and household ornamental flowers (US Environmental Protection Agency, 1973). A residue tolerance of 7 mg/kg, calculated as zinc ethylenebisdithiocarbamate, has been established in the US on about 50 raw agricultural commodities (US Code of Federal Regulations, 1974).

Ziram is also used in the rubber-processing industry as an accelerator or promoter which functions by interacting with sulphur to increase the rate of vulcanization (Wolfe, 1971).

Small amounts are used in industrial fungicides, in combination with 2-mercaptobenzothiazole, in adhesives (including those used in food packaging), paper coatings (for non-food contact), industrial cooling water, latex-coated articles, neoprene, paper and paperboard, plastics (polyethylene and poly-styrene) and textiles (US Environmental Protection Agency, 1973).

In December 1974, the Joint Meeting of the FAO Working Party of Experts on Pesticide Residues and the WHO Expert Committee on Pesticide Residues established a revised temporary acceptable daily intake for man of 0-0.005 mg/kg bw for all dithiocarbamate fungicides (WHO, 1975a,b).

2.2 Occurrence

Ziram is not known to occur as a natural product.

As part of the 'Total Diet Program' of the US Food and Drug Administration, 360 composite food samples were collected annually during the period 1964-1970, prepared as for consumption and analysed for dithiocarbamate content. A maximum of 4 composites contained detectable levels of dithio-carbamates in any single year (Corneliussen, 1972), and in at least one year no dithiocarbamate was detected. On the basis of these results, analysis for dithiocarbamates in this programme was discontinued after 1970 (Manske & Corneliussen, 1974).

2.3 Analysis

Methods for the chromatographic analysis of carbamates, including ziram, have been reviewed (Fishbein & Zielinski, 1967).

Gas chromatography has been used to determine ziram residues in food samples (McLeod & McCully, 1969). Thin-layer chromatographic methods have been described in which the presence of ziram was shown by spraying with a sodium azide-iodine reagent (Klisenko & Vekshtein, 1973a) or with cupric chloride hydroxylamine (Fishbein, 1975). In another method, ziram was hydrolysed and the products reacted to yield strongly fluorescent derivatives (van Hoof & Heyndrickx, 1973) which were separated by thin-layer chromatography and visualized under ultra-violet light. This procedure was capable of demonstrating the presence of 20 ng ziram.

Methods for the detection of ziram based on polarography (Budnikov *et al.*, 1974; Klisenko & Vekshtein, 1973b; Supin *et al.*, 1973) and colorimetry (Rangaswamy *et al.*, 1970) have been described.

3. Biological Data Relevant to the Evaluation of Carcinogenic Risk to Man

3.1 Carcinogenicity and related studies in animals

(a) Oral administration

Mouse: Groups of 18 male and 18 female (C57BL/6xC3H/Anf)F_1 mice and 18 male and 18 female (C57BL/6xAKR)F_1 mice received commercial ziram (m.p. 242-257°C) according to the following schedule: 4.6 mg/kg bw in gelatine at 7 days of age by stomach tube and the same amount (not adjusted for increasing body weight) daily up to 4 weeks of age; subsequently, the mice were given 15 mg ziram per kg of diet. The dose was the maximum tolerated dose for infant and young mice but not necessarily so for adults. The experiment was terminated when the animals were about 78 weeks of age, at which time 15, 18, 17 and 17 mice in the four groups, respectively, were still alive. Tumour incidences were compared with those observed among 79-90 necropsied mice of each sex and strain, which either had been untreated or had received gelatine only: the incidences were not significantly greater (P>0.05) for any tumour type in any sex-strain subgroup or in the combined sexes of either strain (Innes *et al.*, 1969; NTIS, 1968).

Of 82 strain A and 54 C57BL mice given weekly doses of 75 mg/kg bw ziram (purity unspecified) by stomach tube for 20 weeks and killed 6 months after the beginning of the experiment, 42/82 (51%) and 4/54 (7%) developed lung adenomas, compared with 23/54 (43%) and 0/28 controls (Chernov & Khitsenko, 1969) [P>0.05].

Rat: Of 60 random-bred rats given 70 mg/kg bw commercial ziram (90.5% pure) twice weekly in water by stomach tube for up to 22 months, 10 survived 22 months, and 4 developed tumours (2 malignant hepatomas, 2 fibrosarcomas). Among 46 untreated controls still alive at 22 months, 1 developed a fibrosarcoma (Andrianova & Alekseev, 1970) [P<0.01].

Groups of 25 male and 25 female 4-week old Rochester (ex-Wistar) rats were fed diets containing 0, 25, 250 or 2500 mg ziram (purity not specified) per kg of diet for 2 years. The lifespans of both treated and control rats were between 600 and 700 days. Of 11 tumours found in treated rats, 3 malignant tumours of the pituitary and 2 thyroid adenomas occurred in rats given the highest dose; a hyperplastic thyroid was observed in a rat given the lowest dose. Seven tumours were seen in control rats, but their locations were not indicated (Hodge *et al.*, 1956).

(b)   Subcutaneous administration

Mouse: Groups of 18 male and 18 female (C57BL/6xC3H/Anf)F_1 mice and 18 male and 18 female (C57BL/6xAKR)F_1 mice were given single s.c. injections of 46.4 mg/kg bw commercial ziram (m.p. 242-257°C) in 0.5% gelatine on the 28th day of life and were observed until they were about 78 weeks of age, at which time 16, 17, 17 and 13 mice in the four groups, respectively, were still alive. Tumour incidences were compared with those of groups of 141, 154, 161 and 157 untreated or vehicle-injected controls that were necropsied. Incidences were not increased (P>0.05) for any tumour type in any sex-strain subgroup or in the combined sexes of either strain

(NTIS, 1968) [The Working Group noted that a negative result obtained after a single s.c. injection may not be an adequate basis for discounting carcinogenicity].

Rat: Of 48 random-bred rats given 15 mg/kg bw ziram (90.5% pure) in a subcutaneously implanted 250 mg paraffin pellet, 10 survived 22 months, and 3 developed tumours (1 hepatoma, 1 fibrosarcoma and 1 lymphosarcoma of the intestine). No tumours were observed at the site of implantation. Of 46 controls, which did not receive paraffin pellets and which were still alive at 22 months, 1 developed a fibrosarcoma (Andrianova & Alekseev, 1970) [P<0.02].

3.2 Other relevant biological data

(a) Experimental systems

The oral LD_{50} of ziram in rats is 1400 mg/kg bw, and the lethal ranges of oral doses in guinea-pigs and rabbits are 100-150 and 100-1020 mg/kg bw, respectively; dogs tolerated doses of 25 mg/kg bw/day for one month (Hodge *et al.*, 1952), but convulsions occurred in animals given the dose daily for one year (Hodge *et al.*, 1956).

A glycogenolytic response was elicited in rats by an i.p. injection of 10 mg ziram/kg bw (Dailey *et al.*, 1969). Like most dithiocarbamates, ziram induces the accumulation of acetaldehyde in the blood of rats receiving ethanol at the same time (van Logten, 1972).

Administration of ziram with nitrite in aqueous solution to rats by stomach tube led to the formation of detectable amounts of N-nitroso-dimethylamine in the stomach contents 15 minutes later (Eisenbrand *et al.*, 1974).

Little direct work has been done on ziram metabolism (Izmirova, 1972); Izmirova & Marinov (1972) found water-soluble metabolites in the blood, kidneys, livers, ovaries, spleens and thyroids of female rats 24 hours after oral dosing. Unchanged ziram was excreted in the faeces. The presence of water-soluble metabolites indicates the generation of the dimethyldithiocarbamate ion in the stomach after ingestion of ziram; the work of Hodgson *et al.* (1975) on ferbam is therefore relevant.

Administration of 50 mg/kg bw/day to mice for 15 days substantially reduced the fertility and fecundity of the females but did not affect the fertility of males (Ghezzo *et al.*, 1972).

No increase in the number of recessive lethals in *Drosophila melanogaster* was obtained with ziram; however, only 929 chromosomes were tested (Benes & Sram, 1969). Siebert *et al.* (1970) found no significant increase in gene conversion in *Saccharomyces cerevisiae*; metabolic activation systems were not used in these tests. An increased number of chromosome aberrations in metaphases of bone-marrow cells was found in mice treated with 100 mg/kg bw orally (Antonovich *et al.*, 1971).

(b) Man

A fatal case of acute ziram poisoning has been described (Buklan, 1974).

Pilinskaya (1970) reported approximately six times higher frequency of chromosome and chromatid aberrations in metaphases of cultured peripheral lymphocytes from workers handling ziram. Exposure of cultured human peripheral lymphocytes to 0.003 to 0.06 mg/ml of ziram resulted in a dose-dependent increase in the number of chromosome and chromatid aberrations (Pilinskaya, 1971).

For a discussion of the interaction of compounds such as ziram with ethanol in the blood, see 'General Remarks on Carbamates, Thiocarbamates and Carbazides', pp. 28-29.

3.3 Case reports and epidemiological studies

No data were available to the Working Group.

4. Comments on Data Reported and Evaluation

4.1 Animal data

Oral administration of ziram increased the incidence of liver and subcutaneous tumours in one study in rats, with a limited number of surviving animals; its subcutaneous administration induced a lower yield of the same types of tumours. In one study by oral administration in two strains of mice, no carcinogenic effect was observed. A further study by oral administration in rats could not be evaluated due to inadequate reporting. The limited data available do not allow an evaluation of the carcinogenicity of ziram to be made.

Ziram can react with nitrite under mildly acid conditions, simulating those in the human stomach, to form N-nitrosodimethylamine, which has been shown to be carcinogenic in seven animal species (IARC, 1972).

4.2 Human data

No case reports or epidemiological studies were available to the Working Group.

5. References

Andrianova, M.M. & Alekseev, I.V. (1970) On the carcinogenic properties of the pesticides sevine, maneb, ciram and cineb. Vop. Pitan., 29, 71-74

Antonovich, E.A., Chepynoga, O.P., Chernov, O.V., Rjazanova, P.A., Vekshtein, M.S., Martson, V.S., Martson, L.V., Samosh, L.V., Pilinskaya, M.A., Kurinny, L.I., Balin, P.N., Khitsenko, I.I., Zastavnjuk, N.P. & Zaolorozhnaja, N.A. (1971) Toxicity of dithiocarbamates and their fate in warmblooded animals. In: Antonovich, E.A., Bojanovska, A., Engst, P. et al., eds, Proceedings of the Symposium on Toxicology and Analytical Chemistry of Dithiocarbamates, Dubrovnic, 1970, Beograd, pp. 3-20

Benes, V. & Sram, R. (1969) Mutagenic activity of some pesticides in Drosophila melanogaster. Industr. Med. Surg., 38, 50-52

Budnikov, G.K., Toropova, V.F., Ulakhovich, N.A. & Viter, I.P. (1974) Electrochemical behavior of dithiocarbamates on a mercury electrode. III. Polarographic study of fungicides of dithiocarbamate type in organic solvents. Zh. analyt. Khim., 29, 1204-1209

Buklan, A.I. (1974) Acute ziram poisoning. Sud.-med. Ekspert., 17, 51

Chernov, O.V. & Khitsenko, I.I. (1969) Blastomogenic properties of some derivatives of dithiocarbamic acid. Vop. Onkol., 15, 71-74

Corneliussen, P.E. (1972) Pesticide residues in total diet samples. VI. Pest. Monit. J., 5, 313-330

Dailey, R.E., Leavens, C.L. & Walton, M.S. (1969) Effect of certain dimethyldithiocarbamate salts on some intermediates of the glycolytic pathway in vivo. J. agric. Fd Chem., 17, 827-828

Eisenbrand, G., Ungerer, O. & Preussmann, R. (1974) Rapid formation of carcinogenic N-nitrosamines by interaction of nitrite with fungicides derived from dithiocarbamic acid in vitro under simulated gastric conditions and in vivo in the rat stomach. Fd Cosmet. Toxicol., 12, 229-232

Fishbein, L. (1975) Chromatography of Environmental Hazards, Vol. 3, Pesticides, Amsterdam, Elsevier, pp. 676-692

Fishbein, L. & Zielinski, W.L., Jr (1967) Chromatography of carbamates. Chromat. Rev., 9, 37-101

Ghezzo, F., Coradini, L., Guglielmini, C. & Ninfo, V. (1972) L'azione tossica die ditiocarbamati su sistemi enzimatici. Quad. Sclavo Diagn., 8, 485-494

Hodge, H.C., Maynard, E.A., Downs, W., Blanchet, H.J., Jr & Jones, C.K. (1952) Acute and short-term oral toxicity tests of ferric dimethyldithiocarbamate (ferbam) and zinc dimethyldithiocarbamate (ziram). J. Amer. pharm. Ass., 41, 662-665

Hodge, H.C., Maynard, E.A., Downs, W.L., Coye, R.D., Jr & Steadman, L.T. (1956) Chronic oral toxicity of ferric dimethyldithiocarbamate (ferbam) and zinc dimethyldithiocarbamate (ziram). J. Pharmacol. exp. Ther., 118, 174-181

Hodgson, J.R., Hoch, J.C., Castles, T.R., Helton, D.O. & Lee, C.C. (1975) Metabolism and disposition of ferbam in the rat. Toxicol. appl. Pharmacol., 33, 505-513

van Hoof, F. & Heyndrickx, A. (1973) Thin-layer chromatographic-spectro-photofluorimetric methods for the determination of dithio- and thio-carbamates after hydrolysis and coupling with NBD-Cl. Ghent. Rijks-univ. Fac. Landbl. Med., 38, 911-916

IARC (1972) IARC Monographs on the Evaluation of Carcinogenic Risk of Chemicals to Man, 1, Lyon, pp. 95-106

Innes, J.R.M., Ulland, B.M., Valerio, M.G., Petrucelli, L., Fishbein, L., Hart, E.R., Pallotta, A.J., Bates, R.R., Falk, H.L., Gart, J.J., Klein, M., Mitchell, I. & Peters, J. (1969) Bioassay of pesticides and industrial chemicals for tumorigenicity in mice: a preliminary note. J. nat. Cancer Inst., 42, 1101-1114

Izmirova, N. (1972) A study of the water- and chloroform-soluble metabolites of ^{35}S-ziram by means of paper and thin-layer chromatography. Eksp. Med. Morfol., 11, 240-243

Izmirova, N. & Marinov, V. (1972) Distribution and excretion of sulphur-35-labelled ziram (zinc dimethyldithiocarbamate) and its metabolic products 24 hours after oral administration. Eksp. Med. Morfol., 11, 152-156

Japanese Ministry of Agriculture and Forestry (1975) Noyaku Yoran (Agri-cultural Chemicals Annual), 1975, Division of Plant Disease Prevention, Tokyo, Takeo Endo, pp. 17-18, 254, 267-268

Klisenko, M.A. & Vekshtein, M.S. (1973a) Determination of ziram, cuprazin-II, tetramethylthiuram disulfide (TMTD), and their degradation products (tetramethylthiourea, dimethylammonium dimethyldithiocarbamate, and sulfur) in water using thin-layer chromatography. Metody Opred. Pestits. Vode, 1, 60-64

Klisenko, M.A. & Vekshtein, M.S. (1973b) Polarographic determination of residual amounts of fungicide-derivatives of dithiocarbamic acid. Khim. selsk. Khozyarstne, 11, 840-842

van Logten, M.J. (1972) De Dithiocarbamaat-Alcohol-Reactie bij de Rat, Terborg, The Netherlands, Bedrijf FA. Lammers, p. 40

Manske, D.D. & Corneliussen, P.E. (1974) Pesticide residues in total diet samples. VII. Pest. Monit. J., 8, 110-114

McCallan, S.E.A. (1967) History of fungicides. In: Torgeson, D.C., ed. Fungicides, Vol. 1, New York, Academic Press, p. 14

McLeod, H.A. & McCully, K.A. (1969) Head space gas procedure for screening food samples for dithiocarbamate pesticide residues. J. Ass. off. analyt. Chem., 1226-1230

NTIS (National Technical Information Service) (1968) Evaluation of Carcinogenic, Teratogenic and Mutagenic Activities of Selected Pesticides and Industrial Chemicals, Vol. 1, Carcinogenic Study, Washington DC, US Department of Commerce

Pilinskaya, M.A. (1970) Chromosomal aberrations in persons handling ziram under industrial conditions. Genetika, 6, 157-163

Pilinskaya, M.A. (1971) Cytogenetic action of the fungicide ziram in a culture of human lymphocytes in vitro. Genetika, 7, 138-143

Rangaswamy, J.R., Poornima, P. & Majumder, S.K. (1970) Rapid colorimetric method for estimation of ferbam and ziram residues on grains. J. Ass. off. analyt. Chem., 53, 1043-1044

Siebert, D., Zimmermann, F.K. & Lemperle, E. (1970) Genetic effects of fungicides. Mutation Res., 10, 533-543

Stecher, P.G., ed. (1968) The Merck Index, 8th ed., Rahway, NJ, Merck & Co., p. 1131

Supin, G.S., Klisenko, M.A. & Vekshtein, M.S. (1973) Polarographic determination of residual amounts of fungicide as dithiocarbonic acid derivatives. Khim. Sel. Khoz., 11, 840-842

US Code of Federal Regulations (1974) Protection of Environment, Title 40, part. 180.116, Washington DC, US Government Printing Office, p. 249

US Environmental Protection Agency (1973) EPA Compendium of Registered Pesticides, Washington DC, US Government Printing Office, p. I-Z-11-00.01

US Tariff Commission (1945) Synthetic Organic Chemicals, US Production and Sales, 1941-43, Report No. 153, Second Series, Washington DC, US Government Printing Office, p. 118

US Tariff Commission (1949) Synthetic Organic Chemicals, US Production and Sales, 1947, Report No. 162, Second Series, Washington DC, US Government Printing Office, p. 145

WHO (1975a) 1974 Evaluations of some pesticide residues in food. Wld Hlth Org. Pest. Res. Ser., No. 4, pp. 261-262

WHO (1975b) Pesticide residues in food. Report of the 1974 Joint Meeting of the FAO Working Party of Experts on Pesticide Residues and the WHO Expert Committee on Pesticide Residues. Wld Hlth Org. techn. Rep. Ser., No. 574, pp. 26-28

Wolfe, J.R., Jr (1971) Vulcanization. In: Bikalis, N.M., ed., Encyclopedia of Polymer Science and Technology, Vol. 14, New York, Interscience, pp. 740-741, 747-748

SUPPLEMENTARY CORRIGENDA TO VOLUMES 1 - 11

Corrigenda covering Volumes 1 - 6 appeared in Volume 7, others appeared in Volumes 8, 10 and 11. Listed below are further errors that have since been brought to our attention.

Volume 9

p. 251   para 1   line 3   *replace* 112 mg/kg *by* 1112 mg/kg

Volume 10

p. 73   1.3   (c)   *replace* Refractive index: *by* Optical rotation:

p. 200   2.1   line 4   *replace* (+) *by* (±)

Volume 11

p. 116   1.3   (c)   *replace* $19^{\circ}C$ *by* $-19^{\circ}C$

CUMULATIVE INDEX TO IARC MONOGRAPHS ON THE EVALUATION
OF CARCINOGENIC RISK OF CHEMICALS TO MAN

Numbers underlined indicate volume, and numbers in italics indicate
page. References to corrigenda are given in parentheses.

274

Ponceau MX	8,189
Ponceau 3R	8,199
Ponceau SX	8,207
Potassium bis(2-hydroxyethyl)dithiocarbamate	12,183
Progesterone	6,135
1,3-Propane sultone	4,253
Propham	12,189
β-Propiolactone	4,259
n-Propyl carbamate	12,201
Propylene oxide	11,191
Propylthiouracil	7,67
Quintozene (Pentachloronitrobenzene)	5,211
Reserpine	10,217
Retrorsine	10,303
Riddelliine	10,313
Saccharated iron oxide	2,161
Safrole	1,169
	10,231
Scarlet red	8,217
Selenium and selenium compounds	9,245 (corr. 12,271)
Semicarbazide (hydrochloride)	12,209
Seneciphylline	10,319
Senkirkine	10,327
Sodium diethyldithiocarbamate	12,217
Soot, tars and shale oils	3,22
Sterigmatocystin	1,175
	10,245
Streptozotocin	4,221
Styrene oxide	11,201
Sudan I	8,225
Sudan II	8,233
Sudan III	8,241
Sudan brown RR	8,249
Sudan red 7B	8,253